EYE POWER

An Updated Report on Vision Therapy

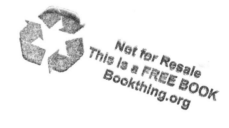
Ann M. Hoopes
Stanley A. Appelbaum, OD, FCOVD

ISBN: 1-4392-2179-0
ISBN-13: 9781439221792
Library of Congress Control Number: 2008911567

Visit www.amazon.com or www.EyePowerBook.com to order additional copies.

In memory of Townsend Hoopes,

who would be so pleased to know that his dream of bringing

vision therapy to the general public is coming closer to being realized.

This book is also dedicated to Barbara, my wife, partner, love and joy of my

life, and to my three remarkable, already accomplished grown up children

whom I adore and admire and make me so proud, give me enormous pleasure,

and help me to never forget what's really important.

Is your child **smart** but totally **frustrated** with school?

Do they **love** to be read to but **hate** to read?

Does **homework** seem to take **forever**?

Are there **tears** with homework?

Is your child **smart** in everything **but** school?

Do they have the diagnosis of ADD, ADHD or dyslexia?

"Eye Power" is for you if you work with or love someone facing any of these challenges!

"Eye Power" is for you if you are searching for answers.

"Eye Power" gives hope, insight and resources to turn frustration into passion and success!

Contents

Endorsements vii

Preface xi

Introduction xiii

Chapter 1
What is Vision Therapy and What Can It Do? 1

Chapter 2
Is It ADHD or Is It Really a Vision Problem? 15

Chapter 3
Kids' Vision and Learning Problems 27

Chapter 4
The Key to Helping Your Autistic Child 39

Chapter 5
From Eyesight to Insight 51

Chapter 6
Vision After a Head Injury or Stroke 71

Chapter 7
Sports and Vision Therapy 89

Chapter 8
Vision Therapy in Action 97

Chapter 9
Lens Therapy 109

Chapter 10
Exercises You Can Try at Home 119

Chapter 11
Nancy's Story 137

Chapter 12
Do You Need Help? 143

Resources 147

Glossary 149

Biographies 155

Index 157

"This is a wonderful, clearly written guide to the many ways that vision therapy can improve how we see and indeed, how we live. There are hopeful clues here to healing attention deficit hyperactivity disorder (ADHD), strokes, and autism as well as to the ordinary problems of vision that beset so many of us. Ann Hoopes, who has been a pioneering educator in the field, quite literally opens our eyes to possibilities of seeing, thinking, and being that have been invisible to most Americans and their physicians."

—James S. Gordon, M.D.
Author
*Unstuck: Your Guide to the
Seven-Stage Journey Out of Depression*
www.jamesgordonmd.com

Founder and Director
The Center for Mind-Body Medicine
5225 Connecticut Avenue, NW, Suite 413
Washington, DC 20015
Tel. (202) 537-6837
www.cmbm.org

"Nothing is more important to us than our vision. *Eye Power* is a fascinating exposition of how, through proper training, we can better see the world around us. Highly recommended!"

—Douglas Brinkley
Author and Distinguished Professor of History
Rice University

History Commentator, CBS News
Contributing Editor, *Vanity Fair* magazine

"During my 30 years of clinical practice as an internist in Bethesda, Maryland, I have had several occasions to share patients with Dr. Appelbaum. I have found vision therapy to be quite helpful in patients with ADD be they young or adults, those who have suffered head injury, in cases of strabismus, and following a stroke. I was initially skeptical that vision training might ameliorate or correct such conditions but have come to learn through experience that this therapy is extremely valuable. Congratulations to Ann Hoopes and Dr. Appelbaum for sharing this important therapy with the public."

—Leonard A. Wisneski, MD, FACP
Clinical Professor of Medicine
George Washington University
Adjunct Professor of Physiology and Biophysics
Georgetown University

"Once again, Ann M. Hoopes has made a significant contribution to broadening public awareness of vision therapy. *Eye Power* originally appeared in 1978, coauthored with her husband, Townsend Hoopes. Their relationship with Dr. Stan Appelbaum, and his willingness to impart his knowledge, has enabled Ann to report on the visual challenges of modern society."

"You will be intrigued by the clinical histories presented here and share in the triumphs of individuals who overcame obstacles borne of medical ignorance or arrogance. In the spirit of books written from a holistic perspective, the information will challenge what you think you know about vision and its influence on emotion, attention, thought, and understanding."

"Vision is so much more than 20/20 eyesight, and after reading this book, you will gain a clearer picture of how deeply vision therapy can change lives. From children over-medicated for ADHD, to persons of any age with physical or conceptual challenges, this book presents realistic hope."

"The pairing of Ann Hoope's writing skills with the clinical insights of Dr. Stan Appelbaum, a highly regarded behavioral optometrist, brings a collaborative passion to the challenge of helping individuals reach their full potential."

—Leonard J. Press, OD, FCOVD, FAAO
Optometric Director, The Vision & Learning Center
Fair Lawn, New Jersey

Endorsements

"This is a brilliant volume.

Clearly written, the authors examine the cutting edge of vision therapy and elucidate the broad impact of vision in our daily functioning, thinking and feeling. The genius of this book is that, while it is sophisticated in perspective, it remains readable throughout. The underlying science is sound, and the case histories are inspiring.

In presenting this material, the authors have done a great service to the public and professional alike. This book is a gem. I will recommend it to my patients."

—Philip J. Cohen, M.D., N.D.

"Eye Power" is a must read.   Dr. Appelbaum and Ann Hoopes are passionate people that will inspire you as they help open doors of insight and help gain answers for those who struggle with ADHD, Autism, Acquired Brain Injury, sports and learning. "Eye Power" can help turn your challenges into success! Enjoy this very easy to read book that can greatly improve your family and friend's quality of life."

—Nancy Torgerson, OD, FCOVD
Alderwood Vision Therapy Center
Lynnwood, Washington

"Eye Power is a must read for any parent who's child is not performing to their potential. The authors have provided a wealth of information along with fascinating stories that make it easy and fun to read about a topic that can be confusing to parents and teachers. With greater understanding, parents will have the tools to help recognize if their child has a vision related learning problem and most importantly what to do to correct the problem! I encourage all parents and teachers who know a child who is struggling to read this book."

Dan L. Fortenbacher, OD, FCOVD
Saint Joseph, MI

"Dr. Appelbaum and Ms. Hoopes have done a terrific job of putting together a consumer-friendly guide to understanding the eyes, the vision process, and vision therapy. Most people still equate good vision with 20/20 vision acuity. In this book the authors do a masterful job of dispelling this common notion in clear understandable language and then give practical and excellent suggestions for techniques anyone can do at home to make their vision more comfortable and efficient. Dr. Appelbaum especially does a good job at letting consumers know when they can work on their own, and when they need to seek professional care.

In all, this book is an invaluable service to the public and especially so to people who suffer from eyestrain as well as those who wish to improve their vision."

Barry Tannen, O.D., FCOVD, FAAO
Director, Vision Therapy and Vision Rehabilitation,
EyeCare Professionals, P.C.
Hamilton, New Jersey

Associate Clinical Professor of Optometry
SUNY/State College of Optometry
New York, New York

Preface

In 1978, my husband and I wrote a book called *Eye Power*. I had been through a major epiphany in my health. Fighting my way back from serum hepatitis and a hysterectomy, and unable to regain my energy, I found vision therapy. To my surprise, I soon learned that the well-being I so badly needed could be tapped from within my visual system. Within nine months of vision therapy, I went through nine progressively weaker pairs of glasses and finally didn't need any at all. This was astounding to me, as I had always been near-sighted and astigmatic. I found myself having a whole new "space relationship" to the world. In other words, my ability to focus on projects, to relate to events, to solve problems, and to make contact with ball sports had transformed. The muscles in my back and neck changed dramatically so that I walked more comfortably. My hips realigned, and I found I could walk 3 or 4 miles a day without any problem.

Because of my excitement, my husband and I decided that everyone in the family including our five children should try vision therapy. We were amazed that each one of us had different positive responses. At this point, we began interviewing other patients to see what dramatic changes they had found. Their stories became the core of *Eye Power*, which was published in 1979 by Alfred A. Knopf.

However, ongoing new information in the optometry field convinced us that our original book needed to be updated. My husband having died, I joined forces with optometrist Dr. Stanley A. Appelbaum, one of the leading authorities on vision therapy, to revise *Eye Power*. I have worked with him for more than 20 years as a patient and to raise awareness of vision therapy, a field that has so much to offer. There are exciting developments in vision therapy, and it is more important than ever to raise public awareness of what is possible.

Recent studies have shown that vision therapy is one of the best solutions for attacking the problems of attention deficit hyperactivity disorder (ADHD). Given the millions of children who have already been prescribed powerful stimulant drugs for ADHD, we must find a better answer. At the very least, we must make more people aware of vision therapy and its benefits. Vision therapy can make a real difference in the ADHD world.

Along with people with ADHD, many people with learning disabilities can benefit. Office workers and students who experience "tension headaches" and eyestrain after long hours in front of a computer screen can benefit. People suffering from a variety of developmental disorders including autism can be helped to improve their visual abilities, not to mention stroke and brain injury victims whose vision has been compromised.

Many seniors are prescribed eyeglasses for reading and computer use, which reduce their awareness of the visual field around them. Thus they can easily fall and often do. Vision therapy helps people improve their eyesight, their vision, and their lives. Almost everyone can benefit, no matter where they are in the "visual clock of life." If you are a person who could benefit by some rehabilitation, vision therapy has much to offer. If you are interested in superior health, vision therapy is a key factor in achieving that potential. I can only point to my own history.

In my own life, I have experienced the difference in brainpower when my eyes are working well and together as a team. My friends wonder how I devour books so easily, how I read menus and drive without glasses, participate in sports without glasses, travel with tremendous energy, lead an active social life with many activities in the day and the evening, sleep 7 hours well, and feel thoroughly engaged in life. The answer is that vision therapy has helped me so much in times of tremendous stress. I feel I have a core of strength that I can rely on within myself. It's almost a spiritual experience to feel that I am operating at my best potential. Dr. Appelbaum and I believe it is imperative to spread the word about the effects of vision therapy on brain activity. You can enhance your eye power just as I have!

—Ann M. Hoopes

Eye Power:
An Updated Report on Vision Therapy

It is hard to believe that 30 years have passed since Ann and Townsend Hoopes authored *Eye Power*, the first book written for the public by patients who benefited from vision therapy. That publication proved to be a significant contribution to the understanding of visual function and its implications. And the perspectives offered by Ann and Townsend pave the way for others to share their experiences.

Take note of the dedication of this updated volume by Ann to the memory of her husband, Townsend, and his dream of bringing vision therapy to the general public. Since the appearance of *Eye Power* in the late 1970s, significant organizational strides have been made in this direction. The College of Optometrists in Vision Development (www.covd.org) has dedicated itself to elevating awareness of vision therapy. The Optometric Extension Program (www.oep.org) and the American Optometric Association (www.aoa.org) have been instrumental in educating fellow professionals and the public. Parents Active in Vision Education (www.pavevision.org, www.vision3d.com, and www.visionhelp.com) serve as great resources to the public.

All things considered, our field has done well to help spread awareness of vision as a complex function beyond what an eye chart can measure. But works such as the book you hold in your hands relate a much more powerful story than organizations are capable of telling. Doctors understand a lot about optics and disease and behavior, but the visual experience and needs of each patient are unique. This is where the pairing of Ann's writing skills with the clinical insights of Dr. Stanley A. Appelbaum, a highly regarded behavioral optometrist, brings a collaborative passion to the challenge of helping individuals reach their full potential.

In story after story, you will learn about the case histories of people who have been shortchanged by society. Ranging from the child inappropriately labeled as having attention deficit hyperactivity disorder (ADHD) to patients of various ages struggling to succeed, you will see real-life encounters of persons plagued by self-doubt. It is sad to think that so many individuals are never given the opportunity to benefit from the procedures described in this book. But it is heartwarming to read about personal triumphs such as Ann has experienced for herself.

One of the powerful messages in this book is that vision is pervasive; it affects concentration, memory, and emotions. Modern methods in cognitive neuroscience, such as imaging studies of the brain, show how widely distributed networks are that integrate visual abilities with mind and body functions. After reading this book, you will gain a much deeper appreciation for why vision occurs in the brain rather than in the eyes.

You will encounter the unique tools of optometry, lenses, and prisms, enabling effects well beyond clear eyesight and single vision. These are points that frankly, are not understood by all eye doctors. Chances are that the eye doctor you are seeing now may not be conversant with many of the topics in the book. Don't let that discourage or deter you.

Another powerful message in this book is that vision development is a lifelong process. Visual skills can be gained or lost at any age. Modern science has established that there is plasticity in the visual system far beyond the early so-called critical periods of development thought to end before a child began school. Not only is this crucial for treating amblyopia, or "lazy eye" beyond childhood, but to help patients who have lost visual function due to head injury or stroke restore their visual abilities.

I have had the pleasure of interacting with Dr. Appelbaum for many years, and he is one of a cadre of optometrists who have dedicated their careers to helping patients develop and maximize visual performance. It has not always been easy to deliver the level of care that Dr. Appelbaum and his colleagues provide. Story after story contains a common theme of patients who received simplistic advice at best, or misguided advice about the potential role of vision in their day-to-day limitations. If you recognize yourself in any of these stories, or have friends or loved ones that these stories call to mind, I encourage you to look further into the many avenues this book opens.

The 1970s version of *Eye Power* was ahead of its time. This 21st century update includes vital information about help for patients with attention issues, physical challenges, chronic stress from prolonged computer use, and holistic insights into the intimate connection between vision, behavior, and emotions. Through their efforts, Ms. Hoopes and Dr. Appelbaum have made a significant contribution to our understanding of the visual challenges of modern society. The message again, may be ahead of its time, but the simple fact that you are reading this book helps fulfill Townsend Hoopes' dream of bringing vision therapy to the general public. And it is time for that dream to flourish.

—Leonard J. Press, OD, FCOVD, FAAO
Optometric Director, The Vision & Learning Center
Fair Lawn, New Jersey

What Is Vision Therapy and What Can It Do?

You or your child may be one of the thousands of people who have undetected or unresolved vision problems. Perhaps you're the parent of a child diagnosed with attention deficit hyperactivity disorder (ADHD). Or you're a student with "tension headaches." Or an office worker whose long hours in front of a computer screen are straining your eyes. Maybe you'd love to play more tennis but are embarrassed about your poor game.

You or your child may have a problem with basic visual skills—eye focusing, eye coordination, eye movements, visual perception, or information processing.

Millions of people do not realize they have vision problems because they've been told they have good eyesight, or they wear corrective eyeglasses or lenses. They do not realize that eyesight and vision are not the same. That their "ADHD" symptoms, reluctance to read, "tension" headaches, "counting the pages" when they read, fear of driving at night, problems looking people in the eye, or even fidgeting, may well be vision problems, not eyesight problems.

Research indicates that many normal, healthy people have significant undiagnosed vision problems. Vision disorders are the fourth most common disability in the United States. Most vision problems are traditionally treated with eyeglasses, contact lenses, medication, or surgery. But these treatments are not always the answer when you have problems with your basic visual skills. At least 20 percent of normal, healthy children and adults have vision problems that are not eliminated or significantly improved by the traditional treatments.

Vision therapy, a specialized branch of the optometry profession, has much to offer to children and adults whose progress is hindered by vision problems. Problems most of us don't realize we have. Vision therapy develops and improves basic visual skills and abilities, often dramatically. It can help us learn how to control our eye muscles, naturally. It also improves the comfort, ease, and efficiency of our vision and changes how our brain processes or interprets visual information—our "visual thinking."

The ADHD Impasse

Recently, parents of children diagnosed with ADHD have found themselves torn by conflicting opinions, government regulations, and scientific results. For decades, they had been persuaded by teachers, school systems, and the medical establishment into giving their children toxic drugs to make them fit better into classroom and family life. Then in early 2006, the Food and Drug Administration (FDA) issued warnings about the dangers of several commonly prescribed ADHD drugs such as Ritalin because of their possible links to cardiac problems and hallucinations. In February 2007, the FDA issued an alert to parents and patients on the risks of mental and heart problems, including sudden death, for all ADHD drugs. Parents are already well familiar with the day-in-and-day-out issues and side effects of taking these drugs.

Despite all the controversy, doctors still seem at ease in prescribing the drugs. Already stressed with the daily challenges of an inattentive and hyperactive child, parents now don't know where to turn. Adults diagnosed with ADHD have similar frustrations.

I am a school principal, and I have sent nearly a dozen and half students for vision therapy over the past several years. So far, all but one have done much better with their studies after vision therapy. The one student who did not improve quite as much as the others had some learning issues that did improve somewhat with vision therapy, but the depth of the learning issues was much more than vision problems. Some of the parents have taken out low-interest loans from banks in order to pay for vision therapy. Vision therapy is expensive and not always covered by insurance, but the difference that it makes in a child's life is phenomenal. Most parents don't say too much about getting braces for their child's teeth, but vision therapy is more important than braces. Vision therapy can mean the difference between a child growing up "learning disabled" or growing up soaring at the top of his or her class. I have personally witnessed the restored self-esteem that children have after successful vision therapy and their excitement when they realize that they really can read just like their classmates.

—Kathy, a Maryland elementary school principal

These days, we don't seem to care whether our children first walk at 9 months, 12 months, or even 16 to 18 months. We only start worrying about our children's development if they are not walking by age 2. In contrast, in many parts of the country we ask children to start reading on their first day of kindergarten even though **very few of them are "visually ready."** Many developmental optometrists and other specialists cite this as one of the reasons why more children than ever are showing signs of ADHD, learning disabilities, dyslexia, and emotional, behavioral, and motor problems.

Is It *Really* ADHD?

Doctors often diagnose ADHD without looking into other possible causes for the symptoms. What few people realize—including many doctors—is that **most common ADHD symptoms are identical to visual performance problems.** Inattentive behaviors such as making careless mistakes and distractibility, and hyperactive behavior such as fidgeting or interrupting others are just a few of the symptoms of vision problems that match ADHD problems.

Because of this, some people with vision problems are mislabeled as having ADHD. Furthermore, people already diagnosed with ADHD often have undetected problems with basic visual skills—eye focusing, eye coordination, eye movements, and visual perception. For example, if you have a "wandering eye," the right eye might wander while the left eye focuses on an object or a sentence. Because your brain struggles to resolve the different images from the two eyes, you may feel discomfort when looking at things or reading, which in turn reflects itself in your behavior. People may think you have ADHD.

Vision Therapy—A Proven Solution

Vision therapy is a key to treating some people with ADHD. This is not to say that children or adults who truly have ADHD, shouldn't receive the appropriate medical treatment. ADHD is however, a diagnosis of exclusion. Problems in vision, auditory, movement, balance, language, general and emotional health need to be ruled out *before* the diagnosis of ADHD is made.

Research continues to reinforce what vision therapists have known for many years. We now have scientific evidence from the National Institutes of Health (NIH) and other national eye centers. In 2005, a landmark study[1] supported by the National Eye Institute of NIH provided evidence that vision therapy is an effective treatment for a common problem in which the patient has difficulty using both eyes together as a team during close work such as reading or writing. This vision problem is called convergence insufficiency (CI). The research results were published in *Archives of Ophthalmology.* Another 2005 study[2] published in the journal *Strabismus* established a direct link between ADHD and CI. This is one of the first times the relationship identified between these two disorders was published in a well-respected, peer-reviewed medical journal.

The American Optometric Association (AOA) (www.aoa.org) defines vision therapy as follows:

> Vision therapy is a sequence of activities individually prescribed and monitored by the doctor to develop efficient visual skills and processing. It is prescribed after a comprehensive eye examination has been performed and has indicated that vision therapy is an appropriate treatment option. The vision therapy program is based on the results of standardized tests, the needs of the patient, and the patient's signs and symptoms. The use of lenses, filters, occluders, specialized instruments, and computer programs is an integral part of vision therapy.

Who Else Benefits From Vision Therapy?

Almost everyone can benefit from vision therapy, despite the condition of their eyes, eyesight, or their age. Along with people with ADHD, many people with learning disabilities can benefit. Office workers and students who experience "tension headaches" and eyestrain after long hours in front of a computer screen can benefit. People suffering from a variety of disorders and

---

[1] Scheiman M, Mitchell GL, Cotter S, et al. 2005. "A randomized clinical trial of treatments for convergence insufficiency in children." *Archives of Ophthalmology* 123:14-24.
[2] Granet DB, Gomi CF, Ventura R, et al. 2005. "The relationship between convergence insufficiency and ADHD." *Strabismus* 13:163-168.

illnesses can be helped to improve underdeveloped visual skills and abilities. Athletes, both pros and amateurs, who want to play a better game can benefit from vision therapy.

After vision therapy, I'm finally optimistic about my future!

—Lily

In addition, a growing number of us are interested in healthful longevity. Because we use only a small percentage of our brain cells, we are looking for ways to "turn on" more of our brain as we grow older. There are many theories on how to activate the brain's potential, and vision therapy offers exciting possibilities.

What Is Involved in a Vision Therapy Program?

When you undergo a vision therapy program, you are given special training and procedures, along with appropriate lenses, to—

- Prevent vision and eye problems from developing
- Develop your visual skills so you can perform more effectively at school, work, or play
- Enhance your vision for tasks that require sustained visual effort
- Improve vision and eye problems that have already developed

A vision therapy program involves individualized techniques and procedures that are performed under a doctor's direct supervision, generally in the doctor's office, once or twice a week. Patients practice and perfect these procedures at home between office visits.

The Doctor Says

We learn to see. This can be learned well or poorly.

—Samuel Renshaw, PhD

The first step in any vision therapy program is a comprehensive developmental/behavioral vision examination. A qualified optometrist can then advise you as to whether you are a good candidate for vision therapy and whether vision therapy is an appropriate treatment for you.

Many types of specialized equipment are used in vision therapy programs, such as—

- Therapeutic lenses (regulated medical devices)

- Prisms (regulated medical devices)
- Filters
- Occluders or patches
- Electronic targets with timing mechanisms
- Fusion games, cards, blocks, and mazes
- Computer software and hardware
- Balance boards/walking rails and vestibular equipment
- Biofeedback devices

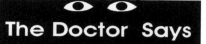

The Doctor Says

In the vision therapy room, I am <u>*the coach*</u> *who raises and lowers the stressors on each procedure so that the trainee (patient) arrives at the "a-ha" response and the new scheme is developed. This is very important to have a coach guide and lead to integrate these schemes."*

—Nancy Torgerson, OD, FCOVD

The program also addresses your nutrition, posture, stress level, and physical condition. A vision therapy program is similar in some ways to training programs for music, football, or the martial arts. Each of these involves discipline and hard work on the part of the trainee, but also requires supervision. There is no other known way to stretch the capacity of the trainee, teach new skills, and raise the level of performance. Vision therapy is not a do-it-yourself program. The doctor is essential as a "coach" during the treatment program.

What Can Vision Therapy Do?

If words looked like this would reading be fun? Would you have to rest your eyes?

Vision therapy develops or improves your basic visual skills and abilities. It also improves the comfort, ease, and efficiency of your eyesight and changes how your brain processes or interprets visual information—your "visual thinking." There are at least 10 common ways in which vision therapy helps:

1. *Improve vision-related reading and learning problems*—The way your eyes move, work together, and focus can affect your ability to read and understand information. Studies have shown that deficiencies in any of these areas can lead to a significant handicap in learning. Vision therapy helps overcome these problems, thereby improving your ability to read and learn. Your ability to visualize in your brain how a printed word looks, enables you to spell that word. If you cannot remember what the word

looks like, you may spell it incorrectly. For example, you may spell it the way it sounds.

2. *Improve skills in visually delayed children*—Vision development is often delayed in children with ADHD, seizure disorders, cerebral palsy, autistic behaviors, or pervasive developmental disorders. Vision therapy is key for helping children build their sensory skills for better learning and function in the activities of daily living.

> *If the key to a better society is education, then the key to a better education is better vision.*
> —Lucy Johnson Nugent
> Daughter of President Lyndon Johnson

3. *Improve vision in "lazy eye"*—Amblyopia, or lazy eye as it is commonly called, is a condition where there is a loss of sight. There are various causes for it. It cannot be corrected even with the best glasses or contact lenses. However, lazy eye is often greatly improved through vision therapy. For many people, lazy eye goes undetected for many years. Studies show **it is never too late to treat a lazy eye**, contrary to what many older doctors still tell their patients.

4. *Improve or decrease cross-eyes or turned eyes*—Strabismus is a condition in which you are unable to align both eyes simultaneously under normal vision conditions. Contrary to common belief, strabismus rarely corrects itself, and children do not outgrow it over time. Cosmetic surgery can sometimes align the eyes more closely. However, by using vision therapy, prisms, and prescription lenses, vision therapy can often help strabismus without surgery. (Even if you have had cosmetic eye muscle surgery, vision therapy is recommended to help improve vision function and depth perception. It is best to have vision therapy before eye muscle surgery to see how much can be improved before surgical intervention.)

5. *Prevent, control, stabilize, or reduce nearsightedness*—Myopia can be controlled safely and effectively for many of us! This is one of the best-kept secrets in health care today. Without the risks and expense of experimental surgery, many people can stop their vision from worsening and in many cases actually reduce their prescription. Techniques include

specialized fitting with modern contact lens materials, reducing eyestrain, improving posture, and nutritional counseling.

6. *Enhance sports performance*—Whether you are a professional or a weekend athlete, vision therapy can give you a competitive edge by improving your depth perception, eye-hand coordination, visual reaction time, dynamic visual acuity, visual accuracy, visual attention, visual anticipation, visual spatial relationships, and visual tracking.

7. *Help after a stroke or brain trauma*—Double vision, headaches, blurred vision, eyestrain, confusion during visual tasks, difficulty reading, visual inattention, visual field deficits, dizziness, vertigo, and balance problems can result after a trauma to the head/brain or a stroke. Vision therapy combined with rehabilitative care can reduce eyestrain, eye fatigue, vertigo, and dizziness, as well as increase independence and balance, reduce symptoms, and enhance the benefits of speech, occupational, and physical therapy.

> *Since I started vision therapy, the only part of me that seems to be getting younger is my eyes!*
>
> **—Donald**

8. *Help children with Pervasive Developmental Disorder, Asperger syndrome, Autistic Spectrum Disorders, and other developmental disabilities*—Vision problems are common with autism and many other developmental disorders, and are often overlooked. Both eyesight and the vision problems need to be addressed. Many common autistic behaviors could be visual problems, such as visual stimulation, "visual stimming," lack of eye contact, looking through or beyond objects, extreme aversion to light, unusual reaction to light, lack of reciprocal play, and inordinate fear of heights or lack of appropriate fear of heights. A visual evaluation by a developmental optometrist may lead to treatment that can positively affect sensory development, sensory integration, and sensory processing.

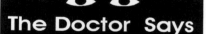

The Doctor Says

When I examine a patient, I ask myself a simple question: "Is the visual system helping or interfering with the patient's ability to achieve his or her potential?"

—Bob Sanet, OD, FCOVD

9. *Alleviate headaches from visual stress*—"Tension" headaches while reading and doing deskwork may be brought on by tired, strained eyes. Vision therapy offers safe, ongoing relief, versus a lifetime of medications and side effects.

10. *Help tired eyes in the workplace*—Even if your workstation is designed correctly and you have 20/20 eyesight and healthy eyes, you may experience blurred or uncomfortable vision when looking at a computer monitor for long periods. These symptoms often result from faulty eye teaming, coordination, and focusing skills. Vision therapy, along with prescription therapeutic lenses, is an effective treatment for these problems.

> **The Doctor Says**
>
> *"You can think of vision therapy as physical therapy for the eye and brain."*
>
> —Carole Hong, OD, FCOVD

What Is Vision Therapy?

Vision therapy is a branch of the optometry profession. Many optometrists who specialize in vision therapy and vision development are educated and board-certified by the College of Optometrists in Vision Development (COVD) and are devoted to developing, improving, and enhancing your visual performance. Vision therapy addresses how the eyes work together with the brain and the rest of the body. It is based on the belief that some eye problems can be improved with techniques that retrain the eyes and the brain to work together better. Thus it uses a holistic approach that addresses your whole system—your eyes, your brain, your mind, and your body.

Aren't "Eyesight" and "Vision" the Same?

The vision therapy profession differentiates between your "eyesight" and your "vision." As Patricia Lemer, M.Ed., explains it, "Eyesight is the sharpness of the image seen by the eye. Vision is the ability to focus on and comprehend that which is seen. Research has shown that while most children with special needs do not have eyesight problems, many have visual dysfunction." Vision is an active process that engages both your brain and your nervous system. Vision is something that you learn to do, to a large degree. Visual problems are at least potentially repairable. Scientists have known for decades that over 80 percent of all learning takes place through the visual system.

Here are some principles of vision therapy:

- Your eyes are not a camera simply recording what is in the environment. Your eyes are receptors of your brain.
- Vision is a complicated and mostly learned process that occurs in your brain.
- From birth, your vision greatly influences the development of your thoughts and personality.

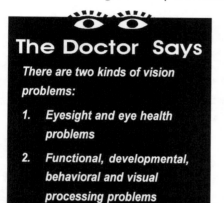

The Doctor Says

There are two kinds of vision problems:

1. *Eyesight and eye health problems*

2. *Functional, developmental, behavioral and visual processing problems*

—Stan Appelbaum, OD, FCOVD

- The building blocks of vision are simple space/time relationships that exist between you and the objects in your field of vision.
- Your ability to locate, interpret, and manipulate physical objects in your field of vision is directly related to your ability to think, create, and solve problems.
- Vision and posture interact. Many visual problems are caused or aggravated by posture problems. Conversely, many posture problems (including backaches and pinched nerves) are caused or aggravated by defective vision.
- Stress affects your visual system, which reduces your energy and constricts performance.

Vision Therapy Isn't Just Eye Exercise

Unlike other forms of exercise that strengthen muscles, vision therapy does not strengthen eye muscles. Your eye muscles are already incredibly strong! In most people, the eye muscles are hundreds of times stronger than they need to be to do anything they need to do. What vision therapy does is help you control your eye muscles and integrate them with all your other senses and visual system. The developmental optometrist believes that your whole body/ mind system will naturally realign itself more harmoniously through effective training and appropriate use of stress-relieving lenses. The result is not only enhanced visual performance but also more energy, better coordination, and greater mental efficiency. You'll be able to see more, do more, and read more, without eyestrain, without working so hard. If you spend too much time doing your homework or your office work, chances are you may be a candidate for vision therapy.

A Typical Visit to Dr. Appelbaum's Office

When I walked into the exam room, I asked Jacob and his mom what had brought them to my office today. Jacob, a third-grader, said "to get my eyes examined," and his mom began to tell me in a very anxious way how Jacob struggles with reading. He loses his place, skips words, reads very slowly, and cries when it is time for homework. The teacher thinks he has ADHD and is recommending medication. Jacob's mom said she recently took him to a pediatric ophthalmologist, who said his "eyes were fine, Jacob has 20/20 vision." She'd made the appointment with me at the urging of Jacob's tutor. The tutor had worked with several of my patients, who were struggling just like Jacob until they started vision therapy. The mom was told that the tutoring went much more smoothly once these kids were able to develop better visual skills and abilities, and some of them no longer even needed to be tutored.

I asked Jacob what were some of the things he liked to do when he had free time, when all his homework was done. I asked where "reading for fun" was on his list. On the top, middle, bottom? Immediately he said "on the bottom." I could see how upset this answer made his mom, who immediately said that she'd recently had Jacob tested by an educational specialist. The results indicated that Jacob was very bright, had way above average IQ, and the recommendation was to put him in a private school with a small class size and extensive tutoring. They had done this, but Jacob continued to struggle. I asked Jacob which were his favorite subjects in school, and he immediately said "math." Was he better at math or reading? He again said "math," which is the classic response for a child with a developmental vision problem.

The Developmental Vision Evaluation that I gave Jacob indicated that the last eye doctor was correct, Jacob had excellent eyesight and healthy eyes, but a very immaturely developed visual system. Jacob's eye movement skills and abilities were at a preschool level even though he was halfway through third grade. He couldn't focus more than a few seconds at a time without rubbing his eyes and complaining of intermittent blurry vision. When I asked if this ever happened in school, he said yes, whenever he read or copied from the chalkboard in school. Jacob had very poor convergence abilities and actually saw two pencils at times when he knew there was really only one pencil. He had not learned how to get his eyes to work together as a team, which is a common problem.

The testing indicated that "stress-reducing lenses" would be helpful for reading and computer use, and we began an office treatment program the following week. After just a few months of vision therapy, Jacob went from a "reluctant reader" to much more of an "avid reader," moving to the top reading group in this class.

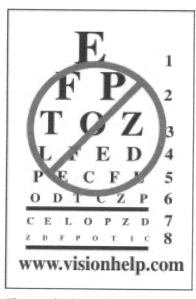

www.visionhelp.com

The standard eye chart does not measure your visual function.

Does 20/20 Eyesight Mean Perfect Vision?

No, 20/20 eyesight does not mean perfect vision; it means at least one of your eyes can see a letter about 1 inch tall from 20 feet away. The 20/20 eyesight test measures how clearly you can see—it does not measure your visual function and does not test your ability to see at closer distances, such as for reading or computer work. It does not tell you if you have headaches with reading, double vision, or visual stamina. The test was created in the 1800s by an eye doctor, Dr. Herman Snellen. This old-fashioned chart also does not evaluate many other important aspects of normal vision such as eye focusing, eye coordination, focus stamina, eye teaming (binocular vision), eye movement, visual perceptual skills, and color vision. This means even though you might not need eyeglasses to see clearly, you still could have a vision problem.

Who Provides Vision Therapy?

The College of Optometrists of Vision Development (COVD) provides board certification in vision therapy to optometrists who have passed oral and written examinations. There is no standard job title for optometrists who practice vision therapy. Depending on where they practice and what kind of patients they treat, these providers may be called optometric vision therapists, behavioral optometrists, developmental optometrists, pediatric optometrists, neuro-optometrists, or functional optometrists. But, in order to be board-certified in vision therapy, they all have passed extensive written and oral examinations by certification boards in vision therapy to demonstrate expertise in this specialty and are referred to as Fellows of the College of Optometrists in Vision Development (FCOVD).

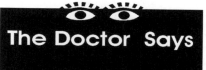

The Doctor Says

Optometrists who provide vision therapy in their offices are called—

- **Developmental optometrists**
- **Behavioral optometrists**
- **Functional optometrists**
- **Neuro-optometrists**
—Stan Appelbaum, OD, FCOVD

Why Didn't My Eye Doctor Tell Me All This?

Your eye doctor may not be aware of vision therapy. Of the approximately 60,000 optometrists practicing in the United States, fewer than 3,000 provide vision therapy. Only about 10 to 20 percent of these doctors have large, full-time vision therapy practices. Vision therapists and regular, traditional eye doctors (optometrists and ophthalmologists) may see your visual defects very differently. The optometrist who specializes in vision therapy believes your visual problems are the result of developmental difficulties, multiple stresses or imbalances in your whole body/mind system. The stresses are caused by factors in your environment or lifestyle. Your vision problem is therefore a changeable condition. Both vision therapists and traditional eye doctors use lenses to treat visual deficiencies, but they use them for different purposes and based on different assumptions. Both groups agree that a patient with healthy eyes who tests at 20/40 on the Snellen test with a typical eyesight problem, could be brought immediately to 20/20 with corrective lenses.

The traditional eye doctor says 20/20 eyesight is possible only when you wear corrective lenses. Some optometrists specializing in vision therapy believe in certain cases, you can achieve 20/20 eyesight without surgery or corrective lenses, through vision therapy and possibly special contact lenses to reshape the cornea (orthokeratology).

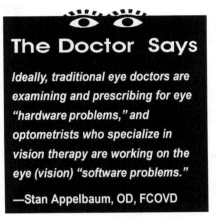

The Doctor Says

Ideally, traditional eye doctors are examining and prescribing for eye "hardware problems," and optometrists who specialize in vision therapy are working on the eye (vision) "software problems."

—Stan Appelbaum, OD, FCOVD

The Doctor Says

Traditional eye doctors examine eyes, Optometrists who specialize in vision problems examine people.

What's the Difference Between the "Three O's"?

Optometrists, opticians, and ophthalmologists are sometimes confused. The Illinois College of Optometry (www.ico.edu) provides a clear description of the roles of these three professions. *Optometrists* examine eyes and prescribe corrective lenses or treatment to protect and improve vision. They are licensed to diagnose and treat vision problems, eye diseases, or other abnormal conditions. They are licensed to prescribe corrective lenses, contact lenses, and other optical aids. Optometrists prescribe vision therapy to remediate, preserve, restore, and improve vision function and efficiency. Some optometrists specialize in areas such as contact lenses, eye disease, low vision, sports vision, or vision therapy. Some specialize in working with children, stroke/brain-injury, ADHD and learning disabilities, or the elderly. *Opticians* are highly trained craftspeople who fabricate and dispense lenses and frames; they do not examine eyes or prescribe treatment. *Ophthalmologists* are licensed physicians who provide medical and surgical care of the eyes.

Dr. Appelbaum Talks About His Patient Diane:

A 33-year-old woman, Diane, came to me for help. She talked about problems getting her work done, being too tired to read her professional journals at night after doing paperwork and e-mails all day, feeling anxious whenever she had to drive at night, and even struggling to judge which step to get on the escalator when she was at the mall, among other complaints. "My eyes are ruining my life," she told me.

She had been to three different doctors, including a highly recommended retina specialist, an eye surgeon, and a neurologist, who found nothing wrong with her eyes and told her no more could be done. She was obsessing over her vision problem and had become unable to think about anything else. She was an anxious person, and this was making her anxiety worse.

When I examined her, with a basic eye health examination, I agreed with the previous doctors that she had 20/20 eyesight and healthy eyes. However, after further specialized testing, my examination indicated that she had binocular instability, (problems getting the eyes to work together as an efficient team), significant problems sustaining focus, intermittent ocular suppression (turning off of an eye by the brain), and convergence insufficiency. We agreed to do vision therapy to try to teach her visual relaxation techniques, how to increase her peripheral awareness, and to gain greater control over her visual skills and abilities.

After just 2 months of office vision therapy, Diane said she was a different woman. Her vision did not bother her as much. She felt as if she could control it. She was amazed at how much happier she had become.

Is It ADHD or Is It Really a Vision Problem?

*"Why can't my son pay attention in school? He's frustrated. . . .
I'm frustrated. . . . And I've tried everything!"*

The Doctor Says

Since the beginning of vision therapy until now, I've seen the greatest change in social areas. Now, he easily and happily joins groups of children.

—Mom

Is your child SMART in everything BUT school? Children who lack good basic visual skills often have a difficult time in school. They enjoy being read to, and will sit and listen, but when they use their eyes for reading and homework, they cannot concentrate. You have tried different methods to help your child, even extra tutoring, but he cannot seem to catch up. Meanwhile, he is getting frustrated and losing self-esteem and may already be feeling a sense of failure.

Your child's teacher may suggest that you get him tested for attention deficit hyperactivity disorder (ADHD). ADHD is a condition that we have all heard plenty about—from parents, teachers, and the media. ADHD is one of the most common behavioral disorders diagnosed in school-age children living in the United States. At least 2 million school-age children have ADHD. Boys are more often diagnosed with ADHD, outnumbering girls more than 3 to 1.

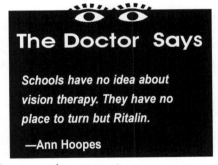

The Doctor Says

Schools have no idea about vision therapy. They have no place to turn but Ritalin.

—Ann Hoopes

ADHD has surged to epidemic proportions in the United States. Consequently, huge numbers of children—

- Are medicated with Ritalin, Adderal, Dexedrine, Concerta, Strattera, and other medications
- Are put into special education classes with special accommodations
- Eventually drop out of school altogether or never reach their potential

Is your child one of these growing numbers? If so, what can you do to help your child?

The usual remedies for ADHD have been to suppress the symptoms with prescription drugs, label children as learning disabled if behavior modification treatment does not work, provide special accommodations such as extra time taking tests, or send children to special education classes. With ADHD presenting a growing threat to children and adolescents, particularly in a culture that emphasizes computers and video games as childhood pastimes, what can you do? According to research published by the *Archives of Ophthalmology* in January 2005, vision therapy is an effective treatment to help these children. For the first time, this landmark study showed conclusively that vision therapy done under direct doctor supervision in an optometric office yields considerably better results than therapy done only at home.

Few people realize that many visual performance problems are identical to the common ADHD symptoms. Because of this, some children with vision problems are mislabeled as having ADHD. Your child's "ADHD" symptoms might very well be an undetected vision problem. In addition, children already diagnosed with ADHD often have undetected vision problems.

In either case, the child may be getting treated with a toxic, psychostimulant drug. In 2006, the Food and Drug Administration (FDA) recommended that several drugs widely used to treat ADHD carry a "black box" warning because they may cause sudden death or serious complications. And in February 2007, the FDA issued an alert on the risks of mental and heart problems, including sudden death, for *all* drugs prescribed for ADHD.

Nobody knows what potential side effects could result from long-term use of these drugs in children. To avoid using such drugs, many desperate parents, as well as teachers and health professionals, are looking for alternative or complementary methods to help children with attention problems or children diagnosed with ADHD. Vision therapy is one such method.

What Exactly Is ADHD?

ADHD is a multifaceted, neurologically based disease. It is not like a germ your child picks up in the playground. According to the most recent version of the *Diagnostic and Statistical Manual of Mental Disorders (DSM-IV-TR),* ADHD consists of three distinct kinds of behavior:

- Inattentive behavior (sometimes called ADD—an outdated term for ADHD)—ADHD inattentive form
- Hyperactive-impulsive behavior—ADHD hyperactive form
- Combination of both inattentive and hyperactive-impulsive behavior— ADHD mixed form

There are children with ADHD who do not have vision problems. **Many ADHD symptoms are identical to symptoms of vision problems. These are the symptoms:**

ADHD Inattention Symptoms
- Does not pay attention to details, or makes careless mistakes
- Has difficulty paying attention during tasks or play activities
- Does not listen when spoken to directly
- Does not follow instructions or does not finish work
- Has difficulty organizing tasks and activities
- Avoids, dislikes, or is reluctant to do tasks requiring sustained mental effort
- Loses things
- Is distracted by outside stimuli
- Is forgetful during daily activities

ADHD Hyperactive-Impulsive Symptoms
- Fidgets with hands or feet, or squirms in seat
- Has difficulty remaining seated when required
- Talks too much
- Answers questions before they have been completed
- Has difficulty waiting his or her turn
- Interrupts or intrudes on others

The Doctor Says

It is vision—not just eyesight— that counts. When the teacher is lecturing, visually competent students are engaged, learning, and creating. Visually incompetent children are not able to use their visual systems effectively so they end up attending to the hum of the air conditioning unit, the tags on their shirts, and the noise in the hall while squirming in their chairs and fiddling with their pencils and paperclips rather than staying visually engaged.

—Stan Appelbaum, OD, FCOVD

— exactly when I had this! ↑

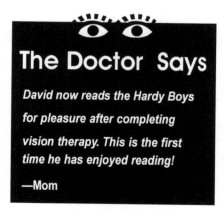

The Doctor Says

ADHD is a diagnosis of exclusion. We need to rule out organic problems such as a brain tumor, sensory integration problems, speech and language problems, and vision problems instead of just using medications.

—Stan Appelbaum, OD, FCOVD

Did you know that a normal child under age 7, at times, has most of the symptoms that are part of an ADHD diagnosis? Furthermore, girls tend not to have the hyperactivity symptoms. It is suspected that girls are also under-identified.

In other words, your child may have the exact same symptoms as those of ADHD, yet many of these problems could be treatable with vision therapy. Even better, your child under 7 with most of the "ADHD" symptoms could be perfectly normal, depending on the severity, intensity, and frequency of symptoms. The key message here is we need to rule out a vision problem if a teacher, parent, or professional suspects ADHD.

The Seven Visual Abilities

Problems with any or all of the following seven visual abilities could be masquerading as ADHD. Vision therapy is used to train all seven of these abilities.

1. 20/20 Eyesight

The best-known visual ability is 20/20 eyesight. Unfortunately, 20/20 eyesight—with or without new glasses—does not mean that during reading and deskwork you can see clearly for more than a few minutes. It does not mean you have the depth perception and localization skills to drive at night or that you are free from vision-caused headaches and general fatigue. 20/20 eyesight simply means you can see clearly long enough to call out six small letters on a doctor's eye chart! Therefore, in addition to 20/20 eyesight, we need six more visual abilities that are generally ignored during routine eye exams.

The Doctor Says

David now reads the Hardy Boys for pleasure after completing vision therapy. This is the first time he has enjoyed reading!

—Mom

2. Eye-Muscle Coordination and Fusion Flexibility and Stamina

The eye has muscles, just like many parts of the body. The brain must coordinate these muscles perfectly so that we can see comfortably and efficiently. Both eyes need to work together even under stressful situations. If this coordination is difficult or off by even a little bit, eyesight may be clear at times and blurred or double at other times. Our unconscious efforts to prevent blurred or double vision can cause premature fatigue, or loss of attention and comprehension during reading, deskwork, and computer work. Some eye-muscle coordination problems can reduce depth perception for driving and sports. Poor eye-muscle coordination can even cause cross-eye or lazy eye.

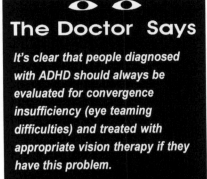

The Doctor Says

It's clear that people diagnosed with ADHD should always be evaluated for convergence insufficiency (eye teaming difficulties) and treated with appropriate vision therapy if they have this problem.

—Stan Appelbaum, OD, FCOVD

3. Eye Control and Focus Stamina

We control our eyes when we maintain eye contact during conversations or keep our eyes on the ball during a soccer game. When our eye control is inaccurate, our vision is inaccurate. It is important to be able to not just get the words clear on the page, but to "keep" the words clear while reading and to change focus quickly and accurately from one distance to another.

4. Visual Tracking and Peripheral Vision

Visual tracking refers to how quickly and accurately we move our eyes across a line of print, look at the symbols (such as numbers, letters, or words), so we can remember what to call them, and get the sounds out of our mouths. Problems with peripheral vision—seeing people and objects "out of the corner of your eye" can reduce peak performance. During reading, children with poor visual tracking lose their place, confuse one word with another, make careless errors, and have difficulty breaking words down into their parts. Prediction plays a significant role in vision. Peripheral vision greatly influences prediction.

5. Visual Perception and Visual Information Processing

Visual perception is our ability to see how things are alike and how they are different, how the pieces fit together to make up the whole. An example is the child who can't see the difference between the letters *b* and *d* or the words, *was* and *saw*. Visual perception problems can make it difficult to recognize words, complete puzzles, do high-level math such as geometry and calculus, or align columns in math.

6. Eye-Hand and Eye-Body Coordination

Our eyes guide, or coordinate, our hands and our bodies. Eye-hand coordination can be "little" or "big." We need "little" (fine motor) eye-hand coordination to copy sentences and to keep words equally spaced and on the line. We need "big" (gross motor) coordination to throw or catch a ball. "Big" coordination is also important for balance and general coordination.

7. Visualization

discussed in PRP handouts

Visualization is sometimes called "seeing with the mind's eye." This means children should "see" words in their minds to spell them and should be able to "see" or imagine (mental movie) a story when they are reading. They can picture their goals in their minds, and the consequences of their actions. Visualization allows us to learn from the past and plan for the future.

Another Example of the ADHD–Vision Connection

According to a study published in 2005 in the medical journal, *Strabismus*, by David Granet, MD, pediatric ophthalmologist at the University of California, San Diego, children with the vision problem convergence insufficiency (CI) are three times more likely to be diagnosed with ADHD than children without the disorder. When you have CI, you have trouble coordinating both eyes together at near distances, such as the distance at which you read. The researchers say CI may be getting misdiagnosed as ADHD, or perhaps ADHD may be causing the CI. In addition, the same problem in the brain that causes ADHD may also cause CI. The researchers also question whether the drugs children take for ADHD may be causing CI.

Dr. Appelbaum Talks About His Patient Nadine:

Nadine was a 12-year-old girl who had had eye muscle surgery because one eye turned all the way inward toward her nose. After the surgery, she had almost constant double vision, and started to need thick glasses. She was finding reading very difficult—she had been reading better before the eye surgery. Her doctor recommended additional eye surgery. Nadine had been diagnosed with ADHD as well and was taking Ritalin.

Nadine began vision therapy twice a week. I had her list some goals: Read longer periods of time, read faster, get rid of double vision or at least have it less frequently, not skip lines or words, not lose her place. She required prism lenses in her bifocals as a result of her eye surgery and was hoping to be able to get out of them. She listed many other additional goals: Be better able to copy from the blackboard. Have to rub her eyes less. Feel less stiff when reading. Be able to see a ball when it's coming. Be able to thread a needle. No dizziness when trying to focus. She hoped her eyes would not be dry and uncomfortable whenever she reads. Nadine wanted to find out why people were so interested in reading. She had never liked reading and wanted to be able to read for pleasure.

The test results showed Nadine was using only one eye at a time. She had almost no binocular, two-eyed, depth perception; she had just enough to cause visual confusion. With her current glasses, she could see almost 20/20 but she could not converge any closer than about 25 inches. Thus anywhere between her nose and 25 inches she was noticing double vision. She hated ball sports, and would not even watch ball sports on TV. It was hard to keep things clear. She noticed problems getting her eyes to work together—one eye would turn inward, and the other would turn outward.

After 2 months of vision therapy, Nadine and her parents commented that she could go a whole school day without double vision and without having headaches. She commented, "When people give me the high five I don't miss anymore." She could keep her eyes straighter. Fewer people would come up to her and say her eyes were not straight. She found it a bit easier to read, even when she was tired.

After 4 months, Nadine's eyes did not wander inward and outward nearly as much. Reading was easier; she could read for longer periods of time, and her grades were improving. She did not have as much double vision when reading or walking around as she used to. She didn't get tired as quickly as before. She discussed coming off of ADHD medication with her doctor and family.

After 6 months of therapy, Nadine was no longer on medication. Her reading had dramatically improved. She was able to keep objects at a distance and nearby, clear and single at the same

continued on next page

Why Does Diagnosis Matter So Much?

A correct diagnosis matters a lot. Many children diagnosed with ADHD are treated with powerful psychostimulant medications. These drugs can cause side effects. A drug frequently prescribed is Ritalin (methylphenidate), a relative of the cocaine family. Common side effects from Ritalin are decreased appetite, insomnia, increased anxiety, and irritability. In addition, stomachaches, headaches, and tics have been reported.

Other drugs commonly prescribed are Dexedrine (dextro-amphetamine), Cylert (pemoline), Adderall (amphetamine-dextroamphetamine), and Strattera (atomoxetine). These drugs also have side effects.

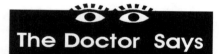

The Doctor Says

Fortunately, we are seeing an increase in schools that recommend that parents of children with vision problems seek evaluation and treatment with a doctor who specializes in vision therapy

—Mark Wright, OD, FCOVD

Some of the drugs can cause visual side effects that actually make it more difficult for a child with ADHD to concentrate on learning tasks. Ritalin and Dexedrine may decrease focusing power or cause dilated pupils and blurry vision. Cylert can cause double vision, eye turns, and nystagmus ("jumpy" eyes). If a child already has one of these visual problems, these medications may actually worsen their problem.

All the drugs may immediately make children more manageable and lengthen the amount of time they spend doing tasks, but often the positive effects do not last. Then the doctor might increase the drug, try another drug, or add a new drug to the current drug. This cycle can continue for years, with new drugs being tried and added. The child can end up taking several powerful drugs at one time. The symptoms return if the child is taken off the drugs, so the doctor may recommend keeping the child on the drugs indefinitely.

Several million children in the United States take Ritalin, Concerta, Adderall, or Strattera every day. The number of children taking medication for attention problems is doubling every 2 years. Production of Ritalin and other medications for attention problems has increased by nearly 500 percent in the last few years.

Where Can I Take My Child for Help?

We believe that a professional clinician who specializes in behavioral conditions—such as a psychiatrist, clinical social worker, or psychologist—is best able to test and observe a child thoroughly to either diagnose ADHD and decide whether medication is absolutely necessary or to help determine that the symptoms are not due to ADHD. These professionals are also trained to rule out other possible behavioral issues. You could also consult a pediatrician, family doctor, or neurologist.

Teachers, school counselors, occupational therapists, physical therapists, speech therapists, and optometrists can recognize the signs and symptoms of ADHD and refer you to one of the above clinicians for appropriate testing.

Unfortunately, many children are being diagnosed too hastily based on parent or teacher recommendations. The clinicians do not determine whether ADHD is the only cause of the symptoms. This often leads to drug prescriptions to handle the problem. As we know, the cause could well be visual.

ADHD is a complex problem. Several specialists should be consulted:
1. Neuro-psychologist, psychologist, and educational specialist
2. Pediatrician or family doctor

3. Occupational therapist
4. Developmental optometrist
5. Speech and language therapist
6. Neurologist

Currently, most parents/patients are relying on one person (specialist) to send them to other specialists. If you have ADHD, you should seek out several specialists simultaneously.

Clinicians dealing with ADHD patients need to become aware of the connection between vision and attention so that they can refer patients to the appropriate doctors, including optometrists specializing in vision therapy, instead of just medicating children with stimulants.

How Can Vision Therapy Help?

Vision therapy improves a child's life. Through different procedures and activities, the doctor and therapist guide the child to help learn how to control his or her eyes and mind to work together. Vision therapy doctors can prescribe a series of special techniques, activities, and treatment procedures to correct problems that glasses alone cannot help.

During vision therapy, the child learns to control eye muscle coordination and builds the vision skills necessary for success in school. Therapeutic lenses are used in a vision therapy treatment program to stimulate visual and overall development, improve visual performance, and reduce visual stress. Therapeutic lenses are based on the understanding of the development of progressive refractive conditions and the fact that sustained near-point activity (reading) is stressful.

We are visually made to do distance activities such as hunting and fishing; we are not made to read. Special lenses are used in vision therapy to reduce the stresses such as when working on a computer or reading a book. These therapeutic lenses are a very powerful tool for patients to immediately alter their perception of the world around them and immediately change how they function in their environment—at school, at home, at work, on the ball field, or driving a car.

Dr. Appelbaum Talks About His Patient John:

John was 8 years old when first seen. His mom was told by the school that they thought he had ADHD. She had him tested, and a psychologist also thought he had ADHD and wanted to put him on medication. The parents were reluctant. His initial issues were squinting, closing or covering one eye when reading or to see better, skipping lines, words swimming on the page, and losing his place when reading. His reading comprehension was poor, and he confused letters, words, and numbers. He confused right and left directions, would make errors copying, and his writing was crooked and poorly spaced. He cried when doing his homework. He read slowly with lots of effort and energy. He had difficulty completing assignments on time. Spelling was a challenge—he would get the words right the night before a spelling test and even do well on the test, but a week or two later he no longer could use the words or spell them. He would complain of seeing more clearly in one eye than the other. He would use his finger as a marker to keep his place and had difficulty remembering what he'd read. He was restless while working at a desk with a lot of inattentiveness and daydreaming. He got very tired at the end of the day especially after completing a visual task. He frequently got carsick. He had problems tracking and moving objects and balls, and his sports performance was inconsistent and poor.

John was seen by an eye doctor who wanted to put an eye patch on him. He was resistant to this. He was diagnosed as having a lazy eye (amblyopia) and was patched most of the day for almost a year. The parents reported little improvement in forcing the poorer seeing eye to see better.

When I examined him, he had a significant difference in eyesight between the two eyes. One eye could see 20/60, and the other was 20/20. There also was a big difference in prescription. When I first saw him, his prescription was three times stronger in the right eye than the left. The right eye was moderately farsighted, and the left was mildly farsighted. During the testing, he commented that the tests made his eyes feel "globby" and "wobbly," and it was hard for him to sustain focus. His eyes were not working together well. When asked to follow an object across his visual field, his whole head moved, and his whole body moved as well. When asked to keep his head and body still, his eyes were jumpy and jerky.

When I first met John, he had "single vision" lenses (as opposed to bifocals), the same lens for both seeing the blackboard and reading. I put him into a bifocal because the testing revealed that his eyes focused differently when he was looking at the blackboard as compared with reading a book. This helped right away. Vision therapy was started twice a week, and John also did activities at home for about 15 minutes a day. Among his parents' goals for the vision therapy were to help him concentrate when reading and when being spoken to, help with his

continued on next page

John's story, continued

handwriting, help with kids' names, making friendships, and relating to other kids better. At recess he was a loner and played by himself. John said he wanted the therapy to help: "I want to stop my eyes from feeling globby. I get tired when I'm reading or listening a lot. I want to do something about that."

After 2 months of vision therapy, John's parents noted the following changes: His reading ability and comprehension were greatly improved; he was more aware of people around him; he did not get distracted as easily and could focus better. He was better at throwing and catching balls. John indicated he could read easier, see letters and numbers, and see TV pictures better because they were "brighter and more comfortable to look at." Remembering was also easier. On the visual memory test at the initial vision therapy evaluation, his standardized test score was barely at a 6-year-old level. After just 2 months of vision therapy, his visual memory score was more age appropriate—at his 8-year-old level.

After completion of vision therapy, John says it's getting more and more easy to read. The letters are bigger now. He says he can see the blackboard better. He also says he is better at finding things. His parents said he now wants to read whenever he has free time, and he has gone up four grade levels in reading. His parents noticed that his personal interactions were better, and he makes eye contact and looks at the person he is talking to for the first time in his life. His parents also commented that he is more confident and aware of the things going on around him, and he is doing better in physical education, such as seeing where the ball goes. John says it's now easier to understand what the teacher is saying, and he can now see out the window. His current teacher is convinced John does not have ADHD and no longer has attention problems.

Kids' Vision and Learning Problems

"Mom, every time I do my homework, my eyes make me feel dizzy!"

Many children have trouble getting their eyes, brains, and body to work together. Unfortunately, over 20 percent of school-aged children have vision problems causing them to struggle to read even though they have 20/20 eyesight. Some of these children suffer from learning disabilities or dyslexia. *Learning disabilities* cause children to have trouble with reading or spelling, writing, and arithmetic. *Dyslexia* is a reading problem caused by the inability of the brain to accurately decode words or phonetically make the connection between the words' written symbols and their appropriate sounds. Reading requires children to accurately use all of their language, decoding, phonetic, and visual skills to successfully recognize words and find meaning in written text.

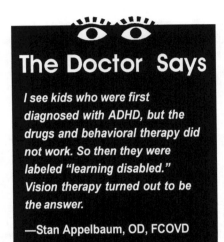

The Doctor Says

I see kids who were first diagnosed with ADHD, but the drugs and behavioral therapy did not work. So then they were labeled "learning disabled." Vision therapy turned out to be the answer.

—Stan Appelbaum, OD, FCOVD

In elementary school, boys are more likely than girls to be diagnosed with learning disabilities. About 20 to 30 percent of children with ADHD have a specific learning disability. However, a large portion of children struggling to read are not dyslexic at all. Their phonetic awareness and language-processing skills may be fine. *Oftentimes, it is their vision that is interfering with their ability to read.* Thousands of children labeled as "learning disabled" actually have correctable problems involving underdeveloped visual skills, eye muscle coordination, or a disconnect between what their eyes see and what registers in their brain.

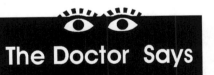

The Doctor Says

Early eye-guided movements of the hand are the "dress rehearsal" for the day when it will be necessary to follow the lines of the printed page.

—Arnold Gesell, MD
  Pediatrician

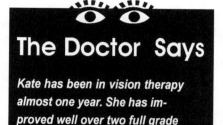

The Doctor Says

Kate has been in vision therapy almost one year. She has improved well over two full grade levels in reading!

—Mom

Vision therapy doctors have known for some time that a significant percentage of children with learning disabilities have some type of vision problem. Recent research corroborates this. For example, many children who are "reading disabled," including those considered dyslexic, have a deficiency in one or more basic visual skills. Yet, teachers and parents often do not make this important connection. As many as one-fourth of all children have a vision problem significant enough to affect their performance in school.

How Important Is Vision to Learning?

Most of our learning in the classroom—an estimated 75 to 90 percent—occurs through the visual system. One out of four children in the United States has some sort of learning problem. This means that millions of students potentially have a vision problem interfering with their progress in school.

Vision is *very often* overlooked by parents and educators as one of the roadblocks a child may be encountering. According to the Better Vision Institute, only 14 percent of children have had a comprehensive vision exam by first grade! Shockingly, in 2005 in the United States, no child could enter kindergarten without having immunization shots; yet only a few states require kindergarten children to have an eye exam. We hope more states will soon follow.

The American Optometric Association recommends that, by first grade, all children should have had at least three vision wellness checkups, one at 6 months, one at 3 years, and again before beginning school, to ensure that their vision is developing on schedule and normally. A thorough vision exam rules out any possible vision problems that may be part of the reason for a child's inappropriate behavior and performance.

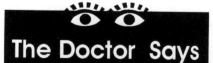

The Doctor Says

Why is vision so important? It's how we connect to the world on an academic, occupational, emotional, and sensori-motor basis

—Curtis R. Baxstrom, OD, FCOVD

20/20 Vision Is Not Enough!

A person's ability to see clearly is called visual acuity. Most people believe that good visual acuity means having 20/20 vision, but having 20/20 vision only means you can see clearly in the *distance*. Schools that conduct vision screenings typically check children's eyesight using a chart across the room (usually a Snellen eye chart). This chart has been used since the Civil War and detects just 20 to 30 percent of vision problems in children! Most schools do not even check children's ability to see up close. Grade-school children tend to be farsighted and not nearsighted. This means they have more difficulty seeing up close than they do far away. It also means that *most children can pass a school vision screening but still have trouble focusing up close, sustaining that focus over a short period of time, or changing their focus quickly from far to near.* Obviously, these skills are essential for activities such as reading efficiently, reading comprehension, and copying from the board.

The Doctor Says

The brighter you are, the more frustrating a problem with your visual system can be. You know that you should be able to do what the other kids are doing. No matter how hard you try, you just can't do as well. People that aren't as intelligent don't notice the difference. Others give up hope and stop trying. You could literally be one of the smartest in your whole school, but no matter how hard you try, you are not able to achieve because vision is getting in the way.

—Nancy Torgerson, OD, FCOVD

However, these skills are only the tip of the vision iceberg! To succeed in school, children must have other important visual skills. They also must be able to—

The Doctor Says

Most kids are brought to me with reading problems when they are in third grade. That's when the print in their school textbooks gets smaller.

—Stan Appelbaum, OD, FCOVD

- Coordinate their eye movements as a team (eye teaming)
- Follow a line of print without losing their place
- Focus clearly as they read or make quick focusing changes when looking up to the blackboard or whiteboard and back to their desks
- Interpret and accurately process what they are seeing

National PTA Resolution

In 1999, the National Parent Teachers Association (PTA) issued a resolution on the importance of educating teachers, parents, administrators, public health officials, and the public about learning-related visual problems. The PTA stressed the need for more comprehensive visual skill tests in school vision-screening programs performed by qualified and trained personnel. In addition, the National PTA urged schools to administer tests for learning-related visual skills needed for success in the classroom in their vision-screening programs. For the full PTA resolution, go to http: www.visionhelp.com/ptaresolution.htm.

Children with inadequate visual skills in any of these areas suffer great difficulty in school, especially in reading. Only a complete vision exam by a developmental optometrist can determine whether vision is the cause of the child's struggle to read.

What Vision Problems Can Be Corrected?

Some symptoms of dyslexia can be corrected if they are the result of a vision problem, such as when the child reverses what he or she sees:

b looks like *d*

was looks like *saw*

p looks like *q*

Another example is the common vision problem, convergence insufficiency (CI), which has several bothersome symptoms that hamper reading:

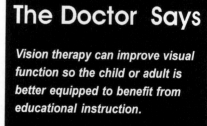

The Doctor Says

Vision therapy can improve visual function so the child or adult is better equipped to benefit from educational instruction.

—Barry Tannen, OD, FCOVD

- Eyes feeling tired or uncomfortable when reading
- Words moving, jumping, or unstable when reading
- Losing your place while reading, or reading slowly
- Suffering eyestrain or fatigue when using a computer
- Only reading when you absolutely have to—thus becoming a "reluctant reader"

A landmark study published in the *Archives of Ophthalmology* in 2005 indicates that vision therapy is the best way to help children with CI.

On October 27, 2008, the Associated Press published an article titled, "Kids Eye Problems Often Emerge in Homework Battle," citing a major government study, finally offers evidence for the best approach: vision therapy in a doctor's office when eyestrain, headaches, double vision, or reading problems trigger the right (visual) diagnosis (CI)."

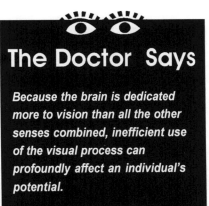

The Doctor Says

Because the brain is dedicated more to vision than all the other senses combined, inefficient use of the visual process can profoundly affect an individual's potential.

—Gary Etting, OD, FCOVD

The National Eye Institute, a division of the National Institutes of Health (NIH) for the U.S. Department of Health and Human Services, released a statement concerning the effectiveness of office-based vision therapy for the treatment of CI. The Convergence Insufficiency Treatment Trial (CITT) published in the October 2008 archives of *Ophthalmology* 126 (10): 1336–1349 found approximately 75 percent of those receiving vision therapy in a doctor's office reported fewer symptoms related to reading and other near work (computers).

The Doctor Says

Children and adults who have visual problems that cause them to read slowly, read only when they have to, or skip words or lines, for the most part have good eyesight. They need vision therapy to "rewrite their visual software programs."

—Stan Appelbaum, OD, FCOVD

These scientific, double blind, placebo-controlled, multicenter studies funded by the NIH are resulting in headlines across the United States such as "New Study Suggests Vision Therapy Is for Real" and "Office-based Treatment Best for Common Childhood Vision Disorder."

How Can Vision Therapy Help?

Parents of children with learning problems should have their children examined by a developmental optometrist to determine whether visual problems exist. Many visual factors can contribute to learning problems. We know that some children have difficulty in school because they are not "visually ready" to learn. If their visual abilities are not

---

Dr. Appelbaum Talks About His Patient Alice:

Alice was in second grade and had a wandering eye. She had seen several eye doctors, one of whom wanted to do surgery, but her mom did not want to do that. The pediatrician referred them to me. When I first met Alice, there were lots of problems. She lost her place when reading, and frequently had to re-read because she could not remember what she had read by the time she got to the bottom of the page and would wonder what she had read. She felt sleepy when reading. She took longer to get her homework done. When reading, she would see the print move or go in and out of focus. She needed directions repeated. She was very quiet and preferred to play alone. She complained of frequent double vision and carsickness, and avoided ball sports. According to her mother, she had intermittent double vision for over 2 years, almost every day. She also had poor posture.

Alice came to me twice a week for treatment. Each session was 1 hour. Her eyesight was 20/20, but I gave her special lenses just for reading and for close work. After 2 months of vision therapy, we did a progress evaluation. Alice and her mom commented that Alice had double vision much less frequently and started to pick up books more. She could now tell when her eyes were seeing double, and do something to correct it; whereas before vision therapy she couldn't. The treatment program continued, and Alice wore her glasses religiously.

After 4 months of vision therapy, the double vision was completely gone, and her eyes appeared straight. She made honor roll for the first time. Her mother reported that the vision therapy home procedures were becoming easier.

A recent progress evaluation showed her double vision was completely gone. She was now a voracious reader. Her mother rarely sees her eyes wandering anymore. She doesn't squint as she used to. She was now in the top reading group in the class. Alice and her mother were thrilled at having avoided surgery to get rid of the double vision.

---

thoroughly evaluated, they may mistakenly be labeled as learning disabled; whereas the underlying problem may be an undetected and untreated vision problem.

Babies are born with eyesight that normally improves as they grow. However, in amblyopia, or "lazy eye," one eye develops appropriately while the other eye continues to see poorly. Amblyopia often goes undetected because a child can see 20/20 with the better seeing eye. Amblyopia is not immediately improved with eyeglasses but is treatable with vision therapy and occlusion (patching) in most cases. It's never too late to treat a lazy eye. Amblyopia vision therapy, as well as the use of the latest vision therapy techniques, has been very successful with adults. If an eye doctor tells you that you are too old to improve your vision in your amblyopic (lazy) eye, it is time to go to another eye doctor who specializes in vision therapy for another opinion.

Strabismus, "cross eyes" or an "eye turn," is seen when you cannot use both eyes together as a team. It can lead to amblyopia, and amblyopia can lead to strabismus because the turned eye fails to develop appropriately. Strabismus can be constant, or intermittent, as when a child is tired. Children with an eye turn may close or cover one eye while reading. They may also squint one eye closed in bright sunlight.

The Doctor Says

Vision therapy is a learning experience that follows a very predictable learning curve. Vision therapy is not eye aerobics. Just like learning to ride a bike, once you learn how to ride a bike, you don't forget how and you don't need to keep practicing to retain bike riding ability—once you learn how to use your vision, you own it.

—Dan Fortenbacher, OD, FCOVD

Treatment for amblyopia or strabismus should begin as early as possible. Early diagnosis and treatment increase the chance for a complete recovery. Current research shows that treatment can be effective at any age. If an eye-teaming problem is left undiagnosed and untreated, for example, it can appear to be a learning disability or dyslexia. It may not be. Eye-teaming disorders are visual problems, not language-based reading dysfunctions. The symptoms, however, are similar.

The Doctor Says

Jamie now has the ability to walk down a moving escalator. Before vision therapy, he was unable to do this. Jamie is now also a better reader as a result of vision therapy.

—Mom

Think of vision therapy as "physical or occupational therapy" for the eyes and brain. Children do not outgrow strabismus or "eye turns." Early detection and treatment are important due to less compensations to "un-do" and more plasticity or flexibility in the system at a younger age. Vision therapy should always be considered as an alternative for strabismus eye surgery. Explore all treatment options, because the success rate is higher for vision therapy than for surgery in many cases of strabismus.

Dr. Appelbaum Talks About His Patient Andrew:

Andrew was a 6-year-old referred by his teacher because he seemed very bright but had difficulty getting his work done in the classroom. The teacher suspected he had ADHD. Both the parents and the child reported he had fatigue with reading, his comprehension dropped with time, and he confused similar words and letters. He held his head close to a book even though he had 20/20 eyesight. While reading, he turned his head and blinked excessively, squinted, and distorted his face. He rubbed his eyes a lot, tilted his head to one side, and turned his head so that he would use one eye only. His sitting posture was poor, and he was restless while working at a desk. He had difficulty copying from the blackboard or a book. His pencil grip was immature. He was confused by directions. He had a short attention span and disliked tasks requiring sustained visual concentration. He frequently displayed signs of frustration when doing close work.

This child had 20/20 eyesight and healthy eyes, having just had an eye exam by a pediatric eye specialist who said his eyes were fine. I found the same, but also found major problems with eye movement control, eye-teaming control, and one of the eyes was being turned off (ocular suppression). Andrew had significant difficulty sustaining focus, problems aligning both eyes, and problems with binocular fusion. When he would try to read, he would break fusion. He complained of intermittent double vision.

I prescribed stress-reducing lenses for close work, to be worn only during reading, writing, and using the computer. He had vision therapy twice a week. Andrew's and his parents' goals were to improve his basketball skills—get 5 out of 10 goals in basketball from 5 or more feet—improve his reading and writing skills, get help with balancing, particularly on one leg, achieve better concentration in schoolwork, and take athletic skills to a higher level.

After 2 months of vision therapy, Andrew and his parents said it was much easier to read the blackboard and follow on a worksheet. He was missing fewer words when reading. He handled the ball better during basketball. His running was increasingly more fluid and faster. He had somewhat better concentration after working on a project, more confidence in reading and drawing, and improved handwriting. He was in a higher reading group in school and didn't have to use his finger as much to keep his place when reading.

After 4 months, Andrew's schoolwork was improving as well as his ability to play basketball. His technique in Tae Kwon Do had significantly improved. His teachers commented to Andrew's parents that they noticed major changes and wondered what vitamins they were now giving Andrew, and what else they were doing to make such dramatic improvements so quickly!

continued on next page

Andrew's story, continued

After 6 months, the parents reported many breakthroughs. He was better able to track work written on the blackboard, left fewer open spaces on worksheets, and now enjoyed reading on his own. His writing skills improved. His eye/hand skills improved so much that he was now on a basketball team and a golf team, and he loved Tae Kwon Do. Testing indicated significant improvements—specifically, visigraph testing and oculomotor testing (an electrographic test in which goggles are put on the patient to enable the doctor to measure where the right eye and left eye are aiming, as the patient reads a paragraph). At the start of vision therapy, there was a huge difference between the two eyes. After 6 months, the two eyes were almost exactly the same.

Finished with treatment, Andrew is now considered the best player on the basketball team. He is better at math and reading. His teacher thinks he is one of the best students in the classroom. His parents are now thinking of switching schools to enroll him in a gifted and talented program.

Many children and adults who have difficulty with reading exhibit abnormal eye movements. The good news is that eye-teaming problems can be treated successfully. CI is an eye-teaming problem usually corrected through vision therapy. Another type of teaming problem called convergence excess can many times be aided with reading glasses and vision therapy. When vision problems are detected and treated, children are more visually prepared to learn in the classroom and at home. Treatment may include more than eyeglasses.

The Doctor Says

Visual processing problems or developmental vision problems can't be detected unless the eye doctor specifically tests for them, which is not part of a routine exam.

—Harvey Mazer, OD, FCOVD

Treatment alternatives include—
- Performance lenses to improve and develop focus flexibility and eye coordination
- Optometric vision therapy to improve visual skills and enhance academic performance
- Visual information processing development procedures
- Prescription eyewear to improve eyesight
- Prism lens therapy to improve spatial awareness
- Visual hygiene suggestions and guidance

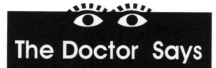

The Doctor Says

We are transforming lives through vision therapy.

—Nancy Torgerson, OD, FCOVD

A program of vision therapy may be needed to develop the visual skills necessary for eye focusing, eye coordination, visual tracking, integration of vision with other senses, and visual information processing. All of these skills are vital to reading and learning.

Dr. Appelbaum Talks About His Patient Aaron:

Aaron is a current patient of mine, age 7, and the son of two elementary school teachers. When he was in kindergarten, his parents first noticed he seemed easily distracted. Nevertheless, he did well that year. "But when he started first grade, he had lost the skills he learned in kindergarten," his mother reported. She said his handwriting was atrocious and he disliked written work. She noted that "he'd rather sit in a corner and cry than do 10 minutes of homework, and we didn't know why." Aaron did manage to stay on grade level that year, however. But over the following summer, he lost the skills he learned in first grade.

Three weeks into second grade, he told his mother, "Mommy, these words make me feel so stupid." By then, the parents suspected dyslexia. They decided to talk to his teacher, who did screenings for special needs. The teacher felt something was wrong because of Aaron's inability to focus and his distractibility. But she said he was not a typical ADHD kid either. Aaron complained that his eyes hurt, and once he said he had blurry vision when reading. He also had problems jumping from the beginning to the end of a sentence and back. The parents decided to take him to an ophthalmologist who specialized in children's vision. During the testing, Aaron was slow at reading the eye chart, and the doctor noted convergence insufficiency (CI). He recommended "pencil pushups" and suggested Aaron wear weak bifocal lenses if the problem did not improve.

In the course of researching CI on the Internet, Aaron's parents came across many references to vision therapy, which they realized they'd heard about as many as 15 years earlier. Wanting to be more proactive in helping Aaron, they decided to give vision therapy a try, and brought him to see me.

After testing, I confirmed the CI and also diagnosed Aaron with intermittent strabismus, visual tracking difficulties, and accommodative dysfunction. I prescribed stress-reducing glasses in

continued on next page

√ I'm getting this,

Aaron's story, continued

the form of bifocals. Aaron began coming twice a week to my office, and doing home activities in between with his parents. After only 4 weeks of therapy, his mother reported that she and her husband were starting to see positive changes.

After 3 months of therapy, she said his whole personality had changed. He was calmer, not so exhausted all the time anymore, and for the first time wakes up happy in the morning. He does not whine as much, and his mother noted that his progress affected the whole family in a positive way. "He now likes to read and be read to, suddenly likes to color, and is better with scissors. He has better hand-eye coordination and is beginning to enjoy physical activities and sports. His schoolwork is now on grade level, and he is no longer struggling so much." Both the parents and I have high hopes that, with progress like this, Aaron's visual skills will be greatly improved by the time he finishes therapy in several months. Aaron used to say he hated school and now he actually enjoys going—a real switch. He no longer cries when doing his homework and works much more independently.

At 4 months, Aaron read his first book on his own. His mom reported that he picked up a "Magic Tree House" book and decided he wanted to read it. Enrolled now in the accelerated reader program at the school, he finished the book, and took the test. The mom reported, "He got seven out of ten right!! Considering it is a 3.5 grade-level book and he is only in second grade, that is pretty good!! This is a kid who hated school and reading 4 months ago!"

The Key to Helping Your Child With Autism

More children than ever before are being diagnosed with autism. If your child is one of them, you, your family, and a team of teachers, doctors, and a host of therapists are working hard to develop your child's abilities. This can add up to numerous appointments and a hectic schedule. In the midst of all of this, you and your support team should know there is another crucial path to pursue—vision therapy. Optometrists who provide vision therapy to patients with autism are called developmental optometrists or behavioral optometrists. They have been helping children with autism lead better lives for some time through vision therapy.

Many people do not realize that people with autism often are held back by severe vision problems. In fact, vision problems manifest themselves in many common autistic behaviors. The patient's eyesight may be "normal," as measured by a standard eye chart test. However, he or she has trouble seeing the world normally: the floor seems to be uneven, objects look blurry, and words move around. This is because the visual system, which receives, integrates, and interprets visual stimuli, is underdeveloped.

In the United States, about one child out of every 150 is now diagnosed with an autism spectrum disorder, according to the Centers for Disease Control and Prevention. This is double the rate of a decade ago and 10 times the rate of a generation ago. Many common autistic behaviors—avoiding eye contact, avoiding looking at the blackboard or whiteboard, poor and uneven handwriting, inability to listen and look simultaneously, flapping hands, walking stiffly, and poking at the sides of the eyes—could be caused by underlying vision problems. Vision problems can sometimes make children and adults behave as if they have mental or physical disorders.

The Doctor Says

Eighty percent of the information we receive comes from the visual sensory system. When we cannot obtain visual information from the environment due to some kind of receptive problem, we then start to see changes in performance or behavior.

—Dr. Melvin Kaplan

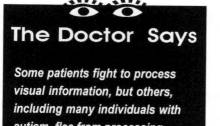

Vision problems often go undiagnosed and untreated in children with disabilities. There are many reasons: perhaps because some believe a visual examination would be difficult, or the child is not able to verbalize a problem, or an eye test has demonstrated 20/20 eyesight.

Vision therapy can have a pivotal role in developmental improvements in a child with autism. Unaddressed vision problems can impair motor development, which then affects social and communication skills. It is important that we do all we can to identify visual problems in children with autism, and begin intervention as early as possible to enable them to reach their full potential.

Vision therapy addresses the underlying visual dysfunctions contributing to many autistic behaviors, using special lenses along with procedures to guide patients with autism to respond more easily to visual information.

What Is Autism?

Scientists have learned much about autism in recent years. It is a dysfunction of the central nervous system that interferes with normal development. The overall scientific name for autism is autism spectrum disorders (ASDs) because scientists believe ASDs are many conditions and syndromes with a wide range of symptoms and severity. Types of ASDs include autism disorder, pervasive developmental disorder (PDD-NOS), and Asperger syndrome. There is a great deal of discussion and controversy about the causes of autism, and researchers are looking at both environmental triggers and genetic factors. Childhood vaccinations, food additives, and pollution have also been blamed. Irregularities in the immune system may have a role, and some studies show that autism can run in families.

Research shows that young children with autism tend to have brains that are larger than normal for their age. Even though they are born with ordinary-size brains, their brains grow considerably by age 2. By age 4, their brains tend to be as large as that of a normal 13-year-old.

The brains of people with autism are "wired" differently too. For example, the visual center in the back of the brain tends to handle tasks usually dealt with in the front of the brain. It is not yet known whether the brain growth and unusual brain activity are basic features of autism or caused by some even more basic problem. The hope is that these abnormalities could be preventable and that early therapy could help normalize the brain.

CDC says as many as 1 in 150 children (or 6 children out of 1,000) have an ASD. Autism is now the sixth most commonly classified disability in the United States. Many children may not be classified as having an ASD until they reach school age or later. Behaviors related to ASDs are usually present before age 3, however, so it is important to identify these children and provide appropriate intervention as early as possible.

What Are the Symptoms?

Symptoms of autism start before a child is 3 years old, even during infancy, and include impaired social interaction and communication, as well as unusual behavior and interests. Children with autism have odd responses to what they see and hear. They can be attracted to some visual stimuli and distressed by others. For example, they often flick their fingers in front of their eyes near a light, staring into the light. They might be oblivious to sound (such as human voices or their own spoken name) or overly sensitive to certain sounds, even very soft sounds. The same child can have both responses. They also may have similar responses to the things they touch, taste, and smell. Their senses can be underresponsive (hypo) or overresponsive (hyper) depending on the day and circumstance.

In our view, some autistic behaviors actually are the child's attempts to view the world while coping with an inadequately developed and poorly integrated visual system. Thus, the child must interact with the world in a simplified or reduced fashion. Many of

The Doctor Says

We combine vision therapy with sensory integration occupational therapy at the same time in our office to get the best results especially with patients diagnosed with an ASD.

—Stan Appelbaum, OD, FCOVD
Barbara Bassin, OTR/L, BCP

these behavior problems can also be seen in children with learning disabilities.

Vision-related symptoms can include—
- Staring trancelike into space, even when walking
- Lack of depth perception
- Looking downward
- Fleeting eye contact
- Tapping toys or making rows of them
- Putting clothes on backwards, or shoes on the wrong feet
- Inability to focus on fast-moving objects
- Not visually attending to sounds or voices

There are many other symptoms, depending on the patient's circumstances.

Recent studies corroborate that the poor eye contact, toe walking, and odd neck and body postures of many people with autism may be attributed to vision problems. Strabismus, amblyopia, and using one eye for far viewing and the other for near viewing are all found in children with autism. In strabismus, or cross-eyed, the eyes do not point in the same direction, which prevents the person from looking with each eye at the same point in space. This can negatively affect depth perception.

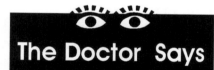

The Doctor Says

Just as language and motor skills are achieved through a sequence of developmental stages, vision must also follow a progression of development.

—Sally Brockett, M.S.

The cause of strabismus can be a disorder in one or both of the eyes, such as nearsightedness or farsightedness, making it impossible for the brain to align the two different images. When the eyes are working independently, rather than together, the patient can see two images instead of one. According to Dr. Melvin Kaplan, 18 to 50 percent of the population with autism suffers from strabismus, compared with approximately 3 to 4 percent of the normal population.[1] Dr. Kaplan's book, *Seeing Through New Eyes: Changing the Lives of Children With Autism,*

---

[1]Kaplan M. 2005. *Seeing through new eyes: Changing the lives of children with autism, Asperger syndrome, and other developmental disabilities through vision therapy.* Jessica Kingsley Publishers.

Dr. Appelbaum Talks About His Patient Larry:

Larry was 7 years old when he started office vision therapy with me. He was referred to me with a diagnosis of autism by his occupational therapist. He also was getting intensive physical and speech therapy. His developmental and fine motor skills were at the 3- to 4-year-old level. Larry did not speak, and he was not reading. When forced to read, he would lose his place and skip words. He had a short attention span, and lots of eyestrain and fatigue when doing close work. He held his head close to the desk or book when doing close work. He disliked tasks requiring visual concentration.

Developmental vision testing indicated that he had healthy eyes and good eyesight (almost 20/20 without glasses). He had major problems getting his eyes to work together as a team and much difficulty with focus stamina. Larry's convergence abilities were very immature, and his binocular skills were unstable. Eye movement control was poor. He had a hard time following a moving object with his eyes alone and had to move his head to follow.

I prescribed stress-reducing lenses for Larry and an office vision therapy program. After 2 months, he showed much less "finger stimulating behavior," and was much less "zoned-out." He engaged in more social interaction with others on the playground, and gave much more attention to reading. Larry was also more comfortable playing soccer. After 6 months of vision therapy, for the first time in his life, Larry would look out the car window at an object passing by. He was finally starting to read. After 8 months, the speech therapist noticed he was finally able to start talking in a meaningful way.

Once vision started to become Larry's dominant learning sense, and his visual skills and abilities started to improve, the speech therapist, occupational and physical therapists all noticed that they were able to get much more out of him during therapy. The occupational therapists started to notice dramatic improvements in his balance and coordination. Larry talked about what he was looking at as he walked around or looked out of the car. After 12 months of vision therapy, he was reading at only a year behind his chronological age and made much better eye contact when talking to parents, teachers, and friends.

Larry tended to look down, so I prescribed glasses for Larry, with special prism lenses to slightly tilt his visual field upward, which helped him look forward rather than down. Vision therapy has improved Larry's reading efficiency and comfort, increased his depth perception, and improved his horizontal and vertical tracking (imperative for math and reading music). Also, Larry's overuse of peripheral vision was improved, which reduced his gaze (and task) avoidance, and decreased the eye poking and other physical signs of visual strain.

Asperger Syndrome, and Other Developmental Disabilities Through Vision Therapy, is an excellent resource for more information.

Amblyopia, or "lazy eye," is characterized by blurry vision not able to be improved with glasses, in an eye that is otherwise physically healthy and normal. People with amblyopia frequently had a period of dysfunction or disuse of their eyes in early childhood during which there was poor transmission of the visual image to the brain. Strabismus can sometimes also cause amblyopia because the brain ignores images transmitted by the "crossed" eye. Another researcher, Dr. Randy Schulman, also found that farsightedness, intermittent strabismus, and other vision problems are frequently encountered in children with autism. Schulman suggested that autistic symptoms such as poor visual pursuit and fixation might be linked to the brain defects reported by autism researchers.[2]

How Can Vision Therapy Help?

Vision therapy helps people with autism lead better lives by addressing any underlying visual dysfunctions that are contributing to the autistic behavior. Vision therapy is a process of training the visual system to function more efficiently. The process involves prescribed activities that are carried out in the developmental optometrist's office and then reinforced with home procedures. Some parents may be told their children's visual problems require surgery. A course of vision therapy often can eliminate the "need" for surgery.

The doctor performs a thorough initial examination to determine what the problems are. The exam includes a series of tests of the patient's ability to see objects at closer distances. No eye drops are used for these "near-point" tests. In the visual evaluation, the doctor may ask the patient to throw and catch a ball, walk up and down stairs, or use scissors to cut along a line. Then the patient puts on special lenses called yoked prism lenses. While wearing different powers of the lenses, the patient repeats the same activities and is evaluated.

---

[2]Schulman RL. 1994. "Optometry's role in the treatment of autism." *Journal of Optometric Vision Development* 25(4): 259–268.

✓ Tell Mark!

Yoked Prism Lenses

Developmental optometrists have had success using yoked prism lenses as a tool for helping children and adults with autism reduce their vision problems. Yoked prism lenses are clear glass lenses slightly thicker on one part of the lens. The lenses bend light in one direction—either up, down, left, or right. They can provide dramatic results by allowing patients to perceive their world differently. For example, glasses with prism lenses might slightly tilt a patient's visual field upward, which helps him or her look forward rather than down.

Dr. Kaplan conducted research in the 1990s that found that vision-related autism symptoms can be reduced with the use of yoked prism lenses. In one study, patients improved in three activities: catching a ball, watching television while seated, and watching television while standing on a balance board. The improvements occurred because by wearing the lenses, patients had more relaxed facial expressions, better posture, and better eye/hand coordination.[3]

These lenses change the electrical activity of the central nervous system. Drugs also affect the nervous system but take five times as long because they involve chemical changes.

The doctor may prescribe yoked prisms for special activities or for full-time wear. The lenses are often an integral part of vision therapy.

The Doctor Says

The use of lenses, which transform light, in combination with visual exercises designed to enable the patient to process visual stimuli in an organized, integrated fashion... can allow the patient to achieve harmony with his environment and reduce the panic responses to visual information that are symptomatic of autism.

—*Dr. Melvin Kaplan*

[3] Kaplan M. 1996. "Postural orientation modifications in autism in response to ambient lenses." *Child Psychiatry and Human Development* 27 (2): 81–91.

Dr. Appelbaum Talks About His Patient Frank:

Frank was 5 years old when he started vision therapy with me. He had been diagnosed by a neurologist to be on the low end of the autistic spectrum.

He had a "funny way of looking at things." He looked with his hands, tilting his head to avoid the use of the right eye. Sometimes he would look at you and other times he wouldn't. Sometimes his eyes seemed half closed. He squinted, and closed or covered one eye when looking at things nearby. When trying to read or copy, he would skip lines, using a finger or marker to keep his place. His writing was crooked, poorly spaced, and illegible. He misaligned letters and numbers. He had great difficulty with, and avoided eye/hand coordination and ball sports such as baseball. Without eyeglasses, his eyesight was 20/30 in the right eye and 20/20 in the left eye.

At home, Frank disliked having his hair and face washed, and his nails trimmed. He avoided certain textures of food. He had difficulty paying attention, and was fidgety and distractible. He was overly sensitive to and distracted by sounds, and needed most directions repeated. He manipulated small objects with great difficulty. He was accident prone, unusually clumsy, and often fell, tripped, and bumped into things. He had poor sitting posture. He had very little language and little interaction with people and with activities.

Upon examination, I found he had a number of vision problems. Frank had a big difference in the retinoscopic reflex between his eyes in spite of the good eyesight in each eye. He had reduced depth perception (stereopsis) and moderate to high esophoria (eyes deviating inward). Testing showed he probably had double vision, yet none had been reported at home or school. These were just some of the problems I observed during examination.

Frank began weekly intensive vision therapy combined with occupational therapy in my office. After 2 months of treatment, his parents reported he was much better at throwing and catching, and had greatly improved in fine motor activities such as printing, cutting, and coloring within the lines. For the first time in his life, he showed significantly less clumsiness in walking and maneuvering.

After 4 months, his ability to concentrate in the classroom had dramatically increased, with a longer attention span for writing and fine motor work. Frank was now markedly less clumsy when navigating around a room or in tight spaces. His printing suddenly was now graded "very good" by the teacher. For the first time, he could copy a shape or word that he was looking at and duplicate something "from sight." After 6 months of office vision therapy, Frank could stick with a task such as building complicated structures with blocks or Legos for long periods. The teacher now said his handwriting was "great... quite an accomplishment from just a few months ago!"

continued on next page

Frank's story, continued

After 8 months of office vision therapy, there were major improvements in Frank's balance, coordination, ability to walk up/down stairs, and running. He was less sensitive to noises and more accepting of transitions. All parts of his body (arms/legs) worked together better, so he had become a really good hitter in baseball and a much happier kid. At Frank's annual visit to the neurologist, the doctor told his parents that Frank had moved up so far in the autistic spectrum, that he was now almost off the spectrum! The neurologist wanted to know all about what Frank had been doing in the past year, and is now referring patients for vision therapy.

An Integrated Solution

Vision therapy can improve reading efficiency, comfort when reading, depth perception, and horizontal and vertical tracking. The use of peripheral vision is reduced, as well as avoiding eye contact, eye poking, and other physical signs of visual strain. Children who have trouble with reciprocal play, such as throwing and catching a ball, oftentimes can soon do much better after vision therapy. If they have an unusual way of walking and refuse to run, these problems often clear up. Overall coordination and alertness are improved, which in turn affects their performance in sports and in school.

It may seem overwhelming to add vision therapy to your already full schedule. But for many people with autism, vision therapy has been the key to significant improvement. They sometimes even say they regret not having started vision therapy much sooner because all other therapies can benefit from adding vision therapy. It's as if vision therapy seems to "open a neurological door" in the brain so that the plateau reached in other therapies can be overcome, and the child can continue to benefit from these therapies. Many times, we recommend starting vision therapy and any other sensory therapies such as occupational therapy before beginning behavioral therapies and interventions to

The Doctor Says

Recognition and utilization of the intricate and complex neurological connection between vision and vestibular function affords a dynamic professional interplay between developmental optometry and occupational therapy, which leads to efficient comprehensive solutions so as to attain optimal patient performance.

—Mary Kawar, M.S., OTR/L

allow your child to later more fully benefit from behavioral therapies and educational instruction.

Through vision therapy, combined with other prescribed therapies, your child's senses can finally start working together. A new book by Patricia Lemer, *Envisioning a Bright Future*, published in 2008, is an excellent resource on interventions that work for children and adults with ASDs.

Combining Vision Therapy With Occupational Therapy

Occupational therapy (OT) addresses areas that interfere with the child's ability to function. Visual skills and abilities are assessed in terms of age-appropriate tasks. OT may be provided to children as play activities to enhance or maintain play, to reinforce self-help, and to improve school-readiness skills. OT benefits a child with autism by attempting to improve his or her quality of life through successful and meaningful sensory motor experiences. OT commonly focuses on improving fine motor skills, or sensory motor skills that include balance (vestibular system), awareness of body position (proprioceptive system), and touch (tactile system).

After the therapist identifies a specific problem, therapy may include sensory integration activities such as massage, firm touch, swinging, and bouncing. Occupational therapists use a variety of theories and treatment approaches when providing services. Many OTs use a combination of approaches when treating children with autism. Combining vision therapy (VT) with OT seems to dramatically enhance the benefits of both therapeutic treatment programs in children with autism.

Many parents have reported positive results with this approach, particularly if OT and VT are done on an intensive basis. Treating patients daily with OT and VT can often result in dramatic improvements in just a few weeks. An article

The Doctor Says

Treatment of visual disorders is a necessary but neglected problem associated with autism spectrum disorders (ASDs) and other developmental disabilities. Hand-flapping, poor eye contact, poor attention, and tantrums are typical and are often caused by vision disorders. Combining vision therapy with occupational therapy in the same office, as we do, results in significant and frequently dramatic benefits.

—Stan Appelbaum, OD, FCOVD
Barbara Bassin, OTR/L, BCP

appearing in the November 18, 2008 edition of the *Washington Post* "Health" section titled, "My son was autistic. Is he still?" says it all. An ongoing study at the Olin Neuropsychiatry Research Center at Hartford Hospital in Connecticut is examining children who once had an autism-spectrum diagnosis, but no longer do. This study has observed that "A growing number of children are apparently emerging from autism and its related disorders to function almost indistinguishably from their peers. . . ."

Recovery from autism is real—something that was unheard of just a few years ago. Utilizing a biomedical approach; dietary modification; nutritional supplementation; detoxification techniques; vision therapy; physical, occupational, and speech therapy; homeopathy; sound-based therapy; and therapies that address communication and social-emotional issues through play have made a dramatic difference in helping the more than one child out of every 150 in the United States on the autistic spectrum. Organizations such as Autism Speaks, and Defeat Autism Now have helped to emphasize early intervention and a hopeful message to parents.

The Doctor Says

Children are frequently referred to an OT for handwriting problems, clumsiness, poor coordination, and difficulty learning. Recent research confirms a high percentage of vision problems in children referred for OT, requiring an evaluation with an optometrist specializing in vision therapy.

—Barbara Bassin, OTR/L, BCP

Dr. Bolar says: Meibomian Gland Dysfunction of my Eyelids — See Dr. Akpek. — Signs of Retina Detatchment, Myopia, Astigmatism, & Presbyopia

From Eyesight to Insight
"Vision therapy is not just for kids."

Are you an adult who feels you're not performing up to your potential? Are you dissatisfied with your vision? There's more to your vision than meets the eye!

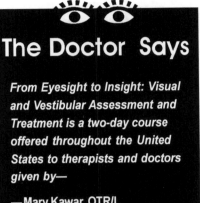

The Doctor Says

From Eyesight to Insight: Visual and Vestibular Assessment and Treatment is a two-day course offered throughout the United States to therapists and doctors given by—

—Mary Kawar, OTR/L
Carl Hillier, OD, FCOVD
Stan Appelbaum, OD, FCOVD

It's not too late to ask yourself whether your vision may be hindering your overall physical and mental performance. Adults with previously undiagnosed visual difficulties or deficiencies can gain improved vision—even exceptional vision— through vision therapy. The benefits are better physical coordination, more energy, greater mental efficiency, and less stress. You have the ability to develop much more control of your performance than you realize. Through vision therapy, you can transform your understanding and your attitude about your eyes. The changes in your life as a result of vision therapy could be profound.

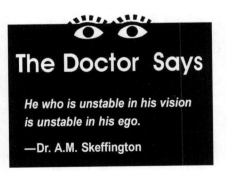

The Doctor Says

He who is unstable in his vision is unstable in his ego.

—Dr. A.M. Skeffington

Even if you've been told you have 20/20 eyesight, you may still be missing critical visual skills. These undiagnosed deficiencies may make learning and reading difficult, disturb your concentration, cause discomfort when you're working at the computer, or be the reason you're constantly tired. Your efforts in college or career may be compromised. Poor posture, stress, driving problems, and difficulty playing sports are also linked to inadequate vision.

Even though it is easier to make changes when we are young, vision therapy benefits adults as well. Research has shown that the adult brain retains a large amount of neural plasticity; unused brain cells can be awakened and put to use. Adult vision therapy patients can improve their brain's ability to use

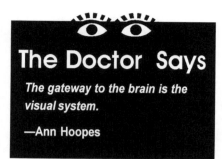

The Doctor Says

The gateway to the brain is the visual system.

—Ann Hoopes

relevant visual information more efficiently through professionally guided repetitive practice. Conditions such as strabismus (poor eye teaming, cross-eye) and amblyopia (lazy eye), particularly, can be improved in adults as well as children.

Vision therapy is not just "eye exercises." When people think about eye exercises, they often think about clear seeing, and the assumption is that the exercises have something to do with eyesight or are an alternative to using glasses or contact lenses. Vision therapy is about much more than *Better Eyesight Without Glasses*, which is the title of a book written by ophthalmologist William Bates, MD, in the early 1940s.

Behavioral optometrists were gratified when renowned physician and author, Oliver Sacks, MD, published an essay in the *New Yorker* magazine in June 2006 chronicling the visual transformation of "Stereo Sue." Dr. Susan Barry, who has a Ph.D. from Princeton University in biology, was born with "crossed eyes," which were straightened through surgery when she was about 2 years old. But during her first 2 years of life—a critical growth period—her brain cells governing three-dimensional vision had not developed because her eyes were not working together.

Dr. Barry did not realize her vision was two-dimensional until she learned while attending college that she had no depth perception. She was still using either one eye or the other. Several decades later, she was referred to a vision therapist, Dr. Theresa Ruggiero, who helped train her vision system to see in "stereo." During 8 months of therapy, Dr. Ruggiero prescribed exercises to improve Dr. Barry's brain's ability to control eye alignment, movements, and visual processing. Dr. Barry described finally seeing three-dimensionally as a thrilling experience second only to the birth of

The Doctor Says

20/20 eyesight does not mean perfect vision. Children and adults with high visual demands often experience visual stress and have undetected visual problems that interfere with their ability to perform, enjoy learning, and become successful and enthusiastic students.

—Carl Hillier, OD, FCOVD

Overall, the changes I have noticed since I began vision therapy are substantially improved distance vision, a great deal of improvement in being able to focus, much less weariness associated with the use of my eyes, and I now actually enjoy "looking," in contrast with before the therapy. I recently told my doctors that I think the only part of me that seems to be getting younger is my eyes, which is really a positive thing for a 59-year-old to say. I actually enjoy the therapy because I can experience the results and follow the progress in a number of the exercises. It is quite impressive. I am still having to work on reading and finding a balance at near distances between my eyes. This remains a challenge, but as I continue vision therapy, I see lots of progress being made here as well.

—Donald

her children. For more information go to: www.oliversack.com/resources.htm and select: "Going Binocular: Susan's First Snowfall."

Vision therapists who work with adults see such transformations all the time. Ann Hoopes is another example. She tells her story below.

Ann's Story

I had worn glasses for near-sightedness and astigmatism from the age of 11 on. When I was 42, I contracted serum hepatitis from a blood transfusion given me during a hysterectomy operation, and the hepatitis subsequently produced a near-total collapse of my health. For the next 3 years, I struggled to get my strength back, with major help from a splendid nutritionist, the late Francis Woidich, M.D. who prescribed no drugs but only diet and vitamins. He put me on a diet consisting chiefly of fresh fruit and vegetables, grain cereal, skim milk, and yogurt, supplemented by large doses of vitamins, with emphasis on A, B, C, and E, plus liver, calcium, magnesium, and potassium. I made steady progress, but my body still suffered from a number of muscular discomforts. One leg was slightly longer than the other, which gave me an uncomfortable hip and back problem, requiring frequent massage therapy for relief. My natural

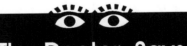

The Doctor Says

With the prevalence of computers in the work environment, we are seeing more adults with eyestrain- related vision problems, which can be improved through vision therapy.

—Neil Draisin, OD, FCOVD

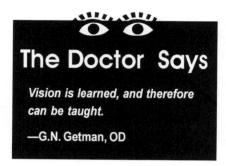

posture was characterized by a slight forward tilt and a very flat back, which seemed to produce chronic upper neck and shoulder discomfort.

Dr. Woidich told me he felt I was losing energy through eyestrain, which compromised his efforts to rebuild my bodily strength. It was true that my energy was still limited, but the idea that I was "losing energy through my eyes" seemed bizarre to me. I had worn glasses intermittently most of my life, but I had never thought much about my vision, except that glasses were a nuisance. Still, I was aware of my increasing need for them.

At Dr. Woidich's suggestion, I went to a behavioral optometrist. He examined my eyes, and then explained to me, in terms I could understand, why I did not see well. My two eyes did not coordinate with each other. I was nearsighted (20/100). Both eyes were astigmatic. I suppressed one eye most of the time. My peripheral vision was weak. When I described to him my various physical ailments, he said they were, in large part, the consequence of my defective vision, and he thought that vision therapy could help correct them, especially my posture problems. I was skeptical, but I was also, at age 42, depressed and frustrated by an accumulation of health problems that were debilitating and apparently insurmountable. Still I could not readily understand how eye exercises could change my body for the better. The doctor said this skepticism was not unusual. He explained the interdependence of vision and posture, and invited me to come to one of his classes and talk to his patients to get an idea of what went on. So I began the therapy.

He told me the training would tend to add some further stress to my already fragile system, and that therefore I would need more sleep than usual. Also, he would want me to undertake a program of physical conditioning with emphasis on walking, jogging, swimming, and calisthenics to build up the cardiovascular system. These activities were necessary to provide a protective cushion against

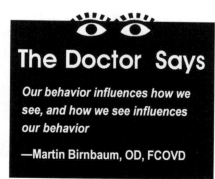

what he called "transitions." I learned that a "transition" in vision therapy is essentially a change from a lower level of visual performance to a higher level. Sometimes it involves a slight shifting of muscles or blood vessels in your neck and upper back, signaling the realignment of your posture with your eyes. At other times it may be a new awareness that your eye-hand coordination has improved. Rarely, a transition is accompanied by temporary physical discomfort.

Each vision therapy session lasted an hour. When I began, my limited energy allowed me to do vision therapy only for about 30 minutes. I did three exercises: (1) walking on an 8-foot balancing rail (4 inches off the ground) while wearing (in rotation) four different pairs of "push-pull" (yoked prism) glasses, (2) tracking with one eye, a small steel ball on the end of a wand that I moved in random patterns, and (3) doing a "divergence-convergence" exercise with a stick while wearing "doubling prism glasses," which cause you to see two of everything. I later learned that these exercises were designed to "disorganize" or shake me out of my existing visual-postural pattern, as a prelude to developing more harmonious eye-mind-body relationships. I also began my physical conditioning regime.

Remarkably, I began to see and feel changes within a few weeks. First I had tingling sensations in my neck and head. Then I noticed that objects farther down the street were in sharper focus, and that my whole visual field was more distinct. The doctor prescribed new glasses for reading and a different pair for driving and distance. After these initial changes, I soon noticed that my old glasses were too strong.

Over one weekend, I experienced a major "transition." Through all of Saturday night, I had the sensation that gears were shifting inside my head; I did not sleep well and awoke with a headache over my left eye, and when I tried to read, there were blank spaces on the page. Sunday morning, noticing that my distance glasses made things look too bright, I took them off and went for a walk. Suddenly I had the sensation of being 8 feet tall, surely the strangest experience I have ever undergone. I was afraid to look straight down at the sidewalk for fear I would topple over, and when I returned home the furniture in the house had shrunk to half its normal size. When I called the doctor, he said, "Well you're having a transition. Go out for another walk or stay home and sleep, but don't read, watch TV, or do anything else with your eyes. Walk to balance out your body with your new visual alignment, or go to sleep." I did both of these things. In 24 hours, the "transition" was over, and I was seeing quite differently. Everything was now consistently brighter and clearer, more intense — the way the world looks in the sudden sunshine after a rain.

The discomfort had been worth it. Now when I looked out the window, the streetlights actually popped out at me. The doctor was pleased to say that, after 40-odd years, I was finally discovering the third dimension. For the first time in my life, I felt actually a part of the scene; whereas before I had always viewed it from outside, as though it were a flatland. Seeing 3-D for the first time was one of the really thrilling moments. I have learned that such new discoveries happen frequently in vision therapy, and that the patient tends to weep or laugh with exhilaration. Some experts call it "critical empathy" — a momentary emotional crisis when you suddenly realize you are seeing things in a new way. Your first reaction is elation. Then you wonder how you could have been locked up for so many years in your old restrictive way of seeing, and you promise yourself to do whatever is necessary to consolidate your new position.

Meanwhile, I was undergoing some interesting body changes. I stood both straighter and more comfortably. The persistent back pain was gone and my legs felt like they were the same length. I was supple enough to sit up and touch my toes, an exercise I had never before been able to do. My astigmatism was almost gone. My eyes worked much more easily together and with far less stress. I was able to drive a car, play tennis, or watch a movie without glasses for the first time in many years. Since then, I wear plus .75 lenses for reading, but no other glasses, and I have more energy.

Over the years since, I have continued to exercise regularly. I get an annual visual checkup with Dr. Stan Appelbaum to determine if any additional office treatment is called for. I am convinced that further improvement—meaning even better, more finely tuned vision—is possible.

Keeping Up in Today's World

The way we are made, is to use our eyes for distance, for hunting and fishing, not for staring at an object within arm's reach for many hours at a time, as most of us do these days. Recent studies indicate that over half of all computer users complain of eyestrain.

When you are working at the computer, your ciliary eye muscles tighten and your extraocular muscles lock into a convergent state, which causes near-point stress. The symptoms are eyestrain, headaches, and double vision. After extended computer use or other close work, your eyes adjust to function more efficiently at close range, and your ability to focus on distant objects is reduced. To correct this problem, millions of us get more powerful glasses to be able to see clearly at a distance. This in turn, makes it more difficult for our eyes to adjust to the computer or to the close work we do, and therefore continues a vicious cycle to stronger and stronger glasses.

I see so well now with my "reduced prescription" glasses after vision therapy, I question the effectiveness of the old stronger prescriptions.

—Marianne

It is not that our eye muscles need strengthening; it is our "brain muscles" that need help. Our eye muscles are actually hundreds of times stronger than they need to be to do almost anything we need to do. It is almost as if people who spend long hours on the computer, complaining of eyestrain, really have "flabby brain muscles."

The Doctor Says

Vision resides in the brain. Any evaluation of the visual system without considering its effects on cognition and movement, is incomplete.

—Carl Hillier, OD, FCOVD

When movement is constrained, the result can be problems like carpal tunnel syndrome from chronic or repetitive stress. Prolonged, concentrated, near activities such as reading, computer use, or too much TV can cause stress on the eye muscles responsible for focusing. This results in an "overload" to the visual system. Traditional eye care frequently means contact lenses and glasses. These provide a crutch and cause dependency but often do not address the underlying problem—an undeveloped visual system that can easily break down with overuse and stress, resulting in fatigue, eyestrain, headaches, avoidance, and underachievement.

Eye-Muscle Coordination

We have six muscles attached to each eye. The brain must coordinate these muscles perfectly so that we can see comfortably and efficiently. If this coordination is difficult, eyesight may be clear at times but blurred or double at other times. Our unconscious efforts to prevent blurred or double vision can cause premature fatigue, or loss of attention and comprehension during reading, deskwork, or computer work. Certain types of eye-muscle coordination problems can reduce depth perception for driving and sports. In extreme cases, poor eye muscle coordination can even cause cross-eye (strabismus) or (amblyopia) lazy eye.

Eye Control

Eye control is used for "keeping our eyes on the ball" or maintaining eye contact during conversations. When eye control is inaccurate, seeing is inaccurate. Our eye control is a direct measure of how vision is affecting our attention. People having trouble looking you in the eye may not necessarily be shy; they may have a correctable eye control problem.

Visual Tracking

We use the term visual tracking to describe how quickly and accurately we move our eyes across a line of print, look at the symbols (such as numbers, letters, or words), remember what to call them, and get the sounds out of our mouths. When reading, poor visual tracking causes a person to lose his or her place on the page, confuse one word with another, make careless errors, and have difficulty breaking words down into their parts.

Visual Perception

Visual perception is the ability to see how things are alike and different, and how the pieces fit together to make up the whole. At one extreme we have the artist who can look at a scene and "see" the relationships between the shapes and colors well enough to reproduce them with paint on canvas. On the other extreme, we have the child who cannot tell the difference between *"b"* and *"d"* or *"was"* and *"saw."* Visual perception problems can make it difficult to recognize words, complete puzzles, enjoy high-level math such as calculus, align columns in math, or—for adults—read a roadmap.

Eye-Hand Coordination

We can divide our ability to get our eyes to guide our hands into "little" (fine motor) coordination and "big" (gross motor) coordination. We need "little" coordination to copy sentences and to keep words equally spaced and on the line. We need "big" coordination to throw or catch a ball or to guide a steering wheel. The "big" (gross motor) type of eye-hand coordination is also very much linked with balance and general coordination.

> *After vision therapy, I'm now able to read for extended periods of time without getting eye fatigue or falling asleep. I can also now wear my sunglasses without eyestrain or tears streaming from my eyes.*
>
> **—John**

Visualization

Visualization is sometimes called "seeing with the mind's eye." If your visualization is good, you can "see" words in your mind to spell them. You can "see" or imagine (mental movie) the story when you're reading. You can picture your goals in your mind. You have the ability to picture the consequences of your actions. Visualization allows you to learn from the past and plan for the future. Reluctant readers oftentimes have poor visualization.

Stress

An extremely important purpose of vision therapy is to reduce physiological stress. Stress is the general wear and tear on the body caused by the body's response to abnormal conditions or demands. Developmental optometrists believe that defective vision is by definition stressful vision, because the mind-body system must use up energy to overcome the defects and achieve enough efficiency to accomplish life's basic tasks.

Intensive near-point vision work such as reading, writing, and working at the computer generates stress, which in turn constricts the visual system. This is both a physical and a mental phenomenon. Even though your eyes do not change structure, and your retina continues to receive as many stimuli as ever, when an eye muscle (or any other muscle in the body) gets tight or loses flexibility because of stress, less information is processed by the eyes and the brain.

The constricting effect of stress on one's visual performance has been demonstrated with a retinoscope. This medical instrument allows the eye doctor to see various levels of light intensity in your eyes, in a variety of situations. For example, when you are relaxed and reading for pleasure at your own pace, the retinoscope reveals a whitish pink color in your pupil. When you are asked to absorb more difficult material but still within your ability to understand, the retinoscope will reveal a true pink color. When you are frustrated by your inability to cope with the material, the retinoscope shows a reddish pink color. Finally, when you give up on the problem, the retinoscope shows a dull brick-red color.

One vision test asks you to begin multiplying in your head two times two, times two, times two. The retinoscope quickly changes color as your mind approaches the frustration and then "wipe-out" level.

Your visual system reacts to stress predominantly in three ways. The first is to develop myopia, which closes out the wider world, but adjusts your mind-body system to cope with a large volume of near-point work. The second is to internalize the stress throughout your various body systems, which leads to a variety of physical ailments, including stiff neck and headache. The third is to drop out entirely (avoidance of reading)—for example, to leave school or quit a job because of your inability to cope with the pressure.

People under stress literally see less, hear less, and become less efficient. Like soldiers, anxious and fearful under the stress of battle, people under stress often develop a "tunnel vision" or a "turn off," leaving them unaware of many aspects of the situation around them.

Vision therapy, by involving not only eye procedures but also activities designed to improve posture, balance, and body awareness is a key to the

Corrine (Age 57) Keeps a Diary During Her First 3 Weeks of Therapy With Dr. Appelbaum:

I was getting more and more nearsighted, suffering from exhaustion, headaches, and watering eyes. I couldn't work at the computer long, and wasn't exercising at all. On my first day of vision therapy, the doctor noted I could see much better with my left eye, but in my right eye the vision was blurred and my depth perception wasn't as good. I was given two exercises to do at home, and told to go for a 45-minute walk.

A great energy lift! On day 3, my vision therapist noticed the depth perception in my right eye still wasn't as good. After two or three repetitions of an exercise with the left eye only, the RIGHT eye got more sharply focused! I saw a difference right away.

The next day, my walk was so enjoyable that I was late for my vision therapy appointment! I noticed that my right eye was in more focus than my left eye, even when beginning the exercises with the right eye. On day 5, my brain recognized its crucial role in vision with the "string exercise," especially with the ring and moving back and forth, and from side to side to keep the ring as one whole image. My brain actually felt as though it had worked very hard. On day 6, I saw improvement in the depth perception in my right eye especially. The next day I was able to relax my focus to bring near objects into focus—"gaze" vision. On day 8, when I worked with the three images—Humpty Dumpty, Old King Kole, and Little Bo Peep—I had a revelation! I felt a sudden change as if a switch was turned on. Then when I got outside I could SEE like I used to! I was practically in tears realizing I could see, I could do this; I could balance things out. It was possible! Tears of gratitude. The doctor explained how to use focusing on the finger to pull the eye in. I had no vision therapy the next day, and walked 45 minutes anyway. My eyes were blurry from computer work until I took the walk.

On day 10, I did some profound work on the 3-D cards: went seven spaces with the card to the right, and could feel my head intensely. I felt the muscles in the back and at the top of my head contract or pull and expand. *Real* physical *work* today! I was too tired to do my eye homework exercises that night. The next day, I did some great work with 3-D images on flip cards. I saw everything as one single image throughout the complete set of cards. On the drive home, I was impressed by my clarity of vision. I worked so hard in vision therapy that I walked 20 minutes afterwards, to process.

On day 12, I had a great session with tracing rings and 3-D glasses. Objects were clearer on the drive home. The next day was cold, and my walk was brisk and invigorating. The doctor complimented me on a good session. I felt solid in my "new vision." On day 14, I learned two new techniques based on older exercises. With the 3-D pictures, I started both pointers at the ocular

continued on next page

Corrine's Story, continued

first. Then with the images of the rings, red and green lenses were added. This was more challenging. I really felt my eyes working. The next morning, I worked 1 hour on the computer. My eyes were feeling tired, and I was making lots of typing mistakes. I started to finish typing just one paragraph, and I began to sense a "headache" appearing. I stopped and jumped up. I ate something and went for a 1½-hour walk. I felt refreshed! On the next day, I had a good vision therapy workout. I found distance vision more challenging during that session and the next day's session. Day 17 was the day of the "stretch"—shifting from near to far vision on the same card. I worked *hard* the next day, and on the following day I worked with the computer for the first time.

On day 20, I found myself reading a number in the telephone book *without* glasses. The number came in and out of focus, but I got it! The next day during vision therapy, I felt my eye and brain muscles truly stretch. Even a snow storm couldn't keep me from going to therapy! I worked with the prism. I felt the eyes strain but much less than last week's prism work. I am so excited to finally feel comfortable when reading and working on the computer and not so exhausted when I come home from work.

relief of stress and to the achievement of higher levels of energy and overall performance.

Who Else Can Benefit?

Behavioral optometrists often work with adults with diagnosed learning problems or ADHD, which we'll discuss below. In addition, people with such conditions as headaches, dizziness, carsickness, vertigo, chronic fatigue, fibromyalgia, or Epstein-Barr syndrome may have an unresolved vision problem. Or if you're too tired to do anything but sit in front of the TV at the end of a day at the office, you, too, should ask yourself whether your vision may be an issue.

Unsteady seniors can have problems getting their eyes to work together. A senior citizen who falls because of an eye-teaming problem is at risk for breaking an arm, leg, or even worse, a hip. Hip replacement surgery is not without considerable risk and can sometimes be prevented by eliminating the reason for the fall—unsteady vision.

How vision therapy improves the vision and lives of adults recovering from brain injuries or stroke is discussed in Chapter 6. Vision therapy for sports enthusiasts is in Chapter 7.

Adult ADHD

If you've been diagnosed with adult attention deficit hyperactivity disorder (ADHD), you certainly should have a vision evaluation and receive vision therapy if necessary. As is the case with children with ADHD, vision problems often go hand in hand with this disorder and are usually unrecognized. Or, vision problems may be masquerading as ADHD.

According to the National Institute of Mental Health (NIMH), ADHD affects approximately 3 to 5 percent of all children, and many will still have it as adults. An estimated 30 to 70 percent of children with ADHD continue to have symptoms as adults. Adults with ADHD often do not realize they have this disorder. They may have trouble getting organized, sticking to a job, or keeping appointments. The everyday tasks of getting up, getting dressed and ready for work, getting to work on time, and being productive on the job can be major challenges for the adult with ADHD.

The Doctor Says

The idea is to assist you in taking charge of your health and to help you create the life you want, rather than simply reacting to the life you have

—Dr. Pete Hilgartner
   Hilgartner Chiropractic Clinic
   Leesburg, VA

To be diagnosed with ADHD, an adult must have symptoms that started in childhood, and the symptoms must be persistent. The diagnosis should be made by a clinician with expertise in the area of attention problems.

As with children, adults with ADHD are often prescribed stimulant drugs—Strattera, Ritalin, or Adderol, among others. In addition, adults may be treated with antidepressants, specifically the tricyclic antidepressants as well as a newer antidepressant, Bupropion (Wellbutrin®). Adults have different concerns regarding ADHD medication than do children. Medication effects may last longer in an adult. Also, an adult may already be taking other medications for physical or emotional problems, such as diabetes, high blood

Dr. Appelbaum Talks About His Patient Joanne:

Joanne was 30 years old and significantly nearsighted, with astigmatism. Her eyes watered whenever she read, and she <u>oftentimes got carsick</u>. She worked at a computer and had intermittent blurry vision and lots of fatigue with reading and focusing on things. She found it hard to remember what she had read. She was unable to work full time because of her vision problem. When she walked, she had to consciously try not to trip. She was an editor, and her work was not very accurate. Her goals were to improve her attention to detail and improve her balance. She was not sleeping well and did not feel rested when she woke up. She wanted to function well even if she slept poorly. In the periphery of her vision, she noticed what she described as "bugs in space" and called "illusory bugs." She would look to the side, and what looked like a bug was not a bug. That is a problem with vitreous floaters and binocular vision. She reported intermittent double vision. Her comprehension decreased the longer she read, and she skipped lines and lost her place on the page. Print would go in and out of focus. Her mind wandered easily when reading. She was restless while working at a desk. Her distance vision blurred when she looked up from close work. She felt nervous, irritable, restless, and frustrated after sustained visual concentration. She found night driving very difficult. Activities that require rhythm were very difficult.

When I tested Joanne, her focusing system was so rigid and tight that even the testing gave her significant discomfort and headaches. The tests revealed that her eyes tended to turn inward (esophoria). She also had right hyperphoria, a tendency of one eye to aim higher than the other. She had very tight fusion ranges, and it was hard for her to maintain fusion—to keep letters clear and single at the same time. She could not converge and keep an object single and clear any closer than 16 inches down her midline. Everything she saw between 16 inches and her nose was seen as intermittent double vision. We found that it was very hard for her to get both eyes to work together as a team. Just wearing her glasses and looking at the small letters on the letter chart, with the right eye covered, the letters were clearer, sharper, blacker, smaller, closer, quicker, easier to see than with her left eye covered. There were big differences between her two eyes that glasses could not fix.

Beginning vision therapy was very difficult for Joanne. The first few sessions made her feel sick to her stomach. She was dizzy, nauseous, and the headaches became worse. She persisted however, continuing with the program. We had her do aerobic exercise every day when she was not in the office.

After 2 months of vision therapy, she noticed that she no longer got nauseated or sick to her stomach when doing any of the vision therapy procedures, either at home or in the office, or in

continued on next page

Joanne's Story, continued

her daily activities. Transitions seem to be easier, going from reading to looking at things far away. Her comprehension started to increase. She found it easier to judge distances. She had slightly less fatigue and more stamina, but not a huge change in the 2 months. The main change was that the therapy was not as difficult to do.

After 4 months of vision therapy, the burning in her eyes was gone. She was able to read for long periods of time. Comprehension and stamina increased. Her headaches were almost completely gone. She found her memory improving, and she <u>seldom got carsick anymore</u>. No more nausea when driving or working on the computer. She said her night blindness had decreased—her ability to drive a car at night is easier. She was less sensitive to light. It was easier to think about things she needed to think about at work.

After 6 months of vision therapy, she had developed more ranges of freedom and flexibility in her focusing system, and in her eye-teaming system. Joanne commented: "I expected to see improvements in how my eyes function, sensitivity to light and motion, difficulty focusing when reading any length of time, difficulty in working on a computer, reading regular-size print and keeping my place there. I wasn't surprised that these things did improve. But what I AM surprised at is that I am <u>not as exhausted during the day</u>. I have so much more energy. What a surprise and delight to see improvements also in my cognitive functions. Many of the tasks that were asked of me in vision therapy were very difficult, but they are becoming easier. I am so happy to see my <u>memory improving</u> and my ability to process information in a normal manner. These are things I had never expected to really develop, and now it seems possible and even likely that I'll be able to function at a high level."

Just over 7 months of vision therapy, and her comments were: "Well, there are so many changes for the better that it's hard to recall them all. Here are some of them: I am now able to work on the computer, maintain visual and mental acuity, drive at night without being blinded by headlights, and remember what I read. Memory has improved dramatically. I have almost no headaches. Sleep is returning to normal. Fewer times of collapse. I'm able to schedule things. And it's now likely my eyes and mind seem to be functioning properly."

After 9 months of vision therapy, Joanne said: "Despite increased stressors in my life I've noticed a greater ability to be aware of what's in the periphery of my vision, sometimes causing a startling response, especially if it's my reflection in a glass door when I know nobody else is around. Words and numbers on the page have settled down so much since beginning vision therapy, while they seem more stable than they were at my last progress evaluation, I am more aware of reading numbers and letters wrong. It seems to happen less often. For the first time

continued on next page

Joanne's Story, continued

since starting vision therapy I've had the experience of proofreading errors leaping off the page. When walking, I look down and I'm in balance and am able to walk smoothly and at a normal pace. I'm able to read notes on a page of music when I'm struggling to determine if each note was above or below the prior one and how many spaces there are below. Piano reading has dramatically improved. Reading comprehension is better. I can work on the computer as long as I need to. Occasionally I'll notice short periods of confusion, but they are less and less often. I almost never get nauseated doing computer work or vision therapy."

With the end of the treatment, most of Joanne's optometric tests were within normal limits. Her convergence is now normal, her focusing is normal, and her eye movement control has dramatically improved as well as her fusion ranges and depth perception.

---

pressure, anxiety, or depression. The ADHD medication could interfere with the efficacy of these drugs.

Your Daily "Visual Hygiene"

Here is a list of tips to get the most out of your vision! The tips are adapted from those provided by Parents Active for Vision Education (PAVE) www.pavevision.org.

- Do all near-point activity at Harmon distance or slightly further. This is the distance from the center of the middle knuckle to the center of the elbow measured on the outside of the arm. Working at the Harmon distance reduces near-point visual stress.
- Be aware of the space between yourself and the page when reading. Also, be aware of things around and beyond the book.
- When reading, occasionally look off at a specific distant object and let its details come into focus. Maintain awareness of other objects and details surrounding it. Do this at least at the end of each page.
- When studying, place a bookmark three or four pages ahead. Get up and move around for at least 1 minute each time you reach the bookmark. Look up, breathe, think about what you are reading or looking at for at least a few seconds, and then continue.

- Sit upright. Practice holding your back appropriately arched while you read and write. Avoid reading while lying on your stomach on the floor. Avoid reading in bed, unless sitting reasonably upright.

- Provide for adequate general balanced lighting, as well as good central lighting, for near tasks. The illumination on the task should be about three times that of the surrounding background. Two lights instead of one are recommended, one light on either side of the working surface, to reduce shadows.

- Tilt the book up about 20 degrees (this slopes up about 4 inches in 12). A tilt top for the desk can be made by screwing two door stops to the back of a piece of ½-inch plywood or a drawing board, and two rubber knobs to the near end so it doesn't slip off the desk. This can be used for reading, studying, writing. It usually enables working farther away from the task than when the task is flat on the desk.

- Do not sit any closer to the television than 6 to 8 feet. Be sure to sit upright and maintain good posture.

- When riding in a vehicle, avoid reading and other near activity. Encourage looking at sights in the distance for interest and identification.

- Do outdoor play or sports activities that require seeing beyond arm's length.

- When outdoors, sight a distant object at about eye level. At the same time, be aware of where things are on all sides.

- Walk with head up and eyes wide open, and look toward, not at, objects.

- Become very conscious of the background of the objects you look toward, be it a person, print on a page, electric sign, the TV, or any other object.

- Try to balance reading, studying, and looking at the computer with aerobic exercise on a daily basis.

- Do the following pumping exercises to work on the ciliary muscles, which are responsible for focusing the eyes' lenses. These exercises help the muscles relax. First, stretch your eyes by rotating both eyes in a circle, first slowly then quickly. Try to make several large circles using your nose as a pointer or pencil. To do the *blur*

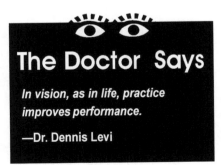

The Doctor Says

In vision, as in life, practice improves performance.

—Dr. Dennis Levi

zoning exercise, focus on the outline of a distant object using your side or peripheral vision until it comes into better focus. For the *fusing exercise*, look closer by crossing your eyes to stare at your nose. These exercises work the extraocular muscles, which move the eyeballs in different directions.

Your "Visual Environment"

I didn't know that I was not seeing the world in 3-D. As I drive through the countryside now, I see that the hills roll and have depth. The trees are not all in the background—some are close and others are far—amazing to perceive it now!

—Judy

When your environment is arranged properly for near-point visual activities such as reading and computer use, the result is reduced stress and improved performance. Research indicates there is a close relationship between posture, working distance, desk surface, and lenses. Beneficial results from experiments by Dr. Darrel Boyd Harmon and later research by Drs. John Pierce and Steven Greenspan included reduced heart rate, more regular and deeper breathing, and reduced neck muscle and overall body tension. To achieve these benefits, the following elements in your environment must be arranged:

- *Working surface:* A sloping working surface—tilted 20 degrees from the horizontal—must be used.
- *Posture:* You should sit comfortably, relatively erect, feet flat on floor or box.
- *Working distance:* The "Harmon Distance" is the optimal distance from the eyes to the working surface. It is the distance from the elbow to the first knuckle. This can only be assured with a proper relationship between your chair height and desk.
- *Therapeutic near-point lenses:* A specific, low-power, doctor prescribed lens should be used, not to correct a defect in the eyes, but to put the eyes into better balance for near tasks. This enhances and integrates the posture, working distance, and working surface relationship.

How Vision Therapy Can Help Adults

The key factors in promoting good visual health are regular eye exercise, appropriate diet and nutrition, low stress, a healthy lifestyle, practicing visual hygiene, and annual vision examinations by an eye doctor who is board

certified in vision therapy. Vision therapy has been
described as a sequential step-by-step stimulation
program to first awaken the quiet pathways in the
brain, which starts the process of using the eyes in
a normal way.

> *Everyone wants an instant
> answer in a pill for whatever is
> wrong. Few people will take the
> time to look for another way.*
>
> **—Ann Hoopes**

Many vision therapists view their work as
"holistic," having seen repeatedly that unrecognized vision problems affect
their patients' well-being, and that behavioral changes affect their patients'
vision. Many vision problems can be traced to early childhood stresses, not to
mention poor nutrition, little exercise, bad posture, improper breathing, lack of
sleep, too much close work, too much time on the computer, and stress later in
life.

Therefore, these optometrists prescribe many kinds of lenses for their patients,
not just those that provide 20/20 eyesight but various others that facilitate
better communication between the eyes and the brain. The result is a
transformation in many areas of their lives, better eyesight and better vision.
Vision therapy in combination with osteopathic treatment, chiropractic
treatment, acupuncture and massage can oftentimes provide dramatic results
in the reduction of symptoms.

Meanwhile, doctors and manufacturers are working on new products and
procedures using computer technology that don't involve glasses, contacts,
drugs, or laser surgery. For example, Dr. Daniel Durrie, an ophthalmologist,
has been testing a technology, developed by NeuroVision, Inc., designed for
patients with mild nearsightedness, or presbyopia, a hardening of the lenses
that makes reading difficult for older people. Dr. Durrie has found that some of
his patients have retrained their brains to focus on images after 30 computer
sessions, each lasting about 25 minutes.

Dr. Peter Shaw-McMinn, an optometrist who has tested more than 70 patients
for neurovision, said adults have more plasticity than researchers realized. He
said, "It was thought that the brain lost neurons with age, and no new neurons
were gained. However, we are able to gain neurons and improve retinal and
visual pathway processing, even as we age."[1]

[1]Passut, J. 2008. Clinical trials reveal promising results for Neuro Adaptation Technology. *Primary Care Optometry News.* April.

In 1992, Dr. Leonard Press, an optometrist in Fair Lawn, New Jersey edited for the Optometric Extension Program a volume titled *Computers and Vision Therapy Programs.* Doctors specializing in vision therapy have been at the forefront of applying technological innovation for their patients.

Computer vision syndrome is one of the fastest-growing health concerns today. Environmental stresses on your visual system (such as excessive computer use or close work) can cause eyestrain, headaches, and/or visual difficulties, which can be effectively treated with corrective lenses and vision therapy. Millions of Americans now use computers regularly. We are becoming an information society, and we are paying the price with our eyesight.

Vision therapy offers the prospect of extraordinary benefit if you are motivated to undertake it. Total performance is the payoff. The basic requirement for success is motivation. Vision therapy is not a quick fix.

Treating your mind/body system as an essential unit can bring improvements beyond visual acuity to posture, muscle coordination, energy, and creativity— and even behavior and personality. Vision therapy has reportedly brought an end not only to blurred vision but also to many other stress-induced conditions due to decreased stress in the whole body. It has strengthened a person's intellectual performance and creativity and at times changed his or her irritable and agitated mental state to one of calmness and self-confidence.

Vision After a Head Injury or Stroke

"Will I ever be able to enjoy reading or drive again?"

Many of us have loved ones who have suffered the consequences of a stroke or brain injury and who are probably still struggling to regain their former abilities. Did you know that people who have experienced a head injury or a stroke are often left with serious vision and eye problems, even after

> *Vision therapy almost "massages" the brain cells to activate them after brain injury.*
>
> **—Ann Hoopes**

they've gone through rehabilitation? They may no longer know where straight ahead is or where things are really located. They get confused at the supermarket or mall. When they read or look around, their eyes land on the wrong spot. They have balance problems, dizziness, carsickness, and possibly double vision. They may not be able to drive anymore. Similar vision-related problems are common in people who have neurological disorders such as epilepsy, cerebral palsy, and multiple sclerosis.

Your loved one could have visual-processing problems and eyesight problems that are not being adequately managed. Neuro-optometrists have long recognized that these problems underlie many of the patient's difficulties, not only with balance and movement but also with his or her perception of space and ability to process this information.

The visual system has a major impact on cognitive and motor function; therefore any visual problems must be addressed as early as possible. The vision problems may be hidden, may have interfered with the rehabilitation, or may have been neglected during the rehabilitation.

Vision therapy that is devoted to vision rehabilitation is called *neuro-optometric rehabilitation*—an individualized treatment regimen that includes the use of special lenses and prisms either with or without occlusion (eye patching), along with optical devices and other appropriate rehabilitation strategies for patients who have had a brain injury, stroke, car accident, and many other neurologic disorders.

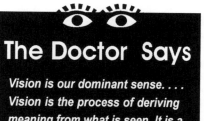

The Doctor Says

Vision is our dominant sense. . . . Vision is the process of deriving meaning from what is seen. It is a complex, learned, and developed set of functions that involve a multitude of skills. Research estimates that 80 to 85 percent of our perception, learning, cognition, and activities are mediated through vision.

—Thomas Politzer, OD,
   Past President, Neuro-
   Optometric Rehabilitation
   Association

Whether it is a head injury, stroke, or neurological disorder, the associated vision problems are caused by injury to nerve pathways in the brain. Vision is made possible through a complex system involving the flow and processing of information to the brain. The visual system perceives an object in space and sends that visual information to the areas in the brain that control movement. Those brain areas command the body to move and then adjust the movements based on sensory and motor feedback.

When the brain is injured, the nerves in the brain and spinal cord (the central nervous system) are stressed. The nerves that control the muscles for eye movements as well as those for the system that regulates focusing may be interrupted. The autonomic nervous system may be affected as well, which regulates all the involuntary activities in the body. Neuro-optometric vision rehabilitation can teach other areas of the brain to take over the functions of the damaged areas.

Research has shown that people of all ages who have experienced neurological vision damage can benefit from neuro-optometric rehabilitation. For example, one study published in the *Archives of Physical Medicine and Rehabilitation* in 1998 found that vision therapy, prisms, and binasal occlusion were helpful in improving binocular integration and double vision from extraocular movement disorders in patients with head injury. The following sections describe some of the ways in which the vision centers in the brain can be injured—through head injury, stroke, and other neurological disorders.

Head Injury

The overall medical term for head injury is traumatic brain injury (TBI), which occurs either when the head hits an object and receives a "closed head injury" or "whiplash," or when something pierces the skull and penetrates the brain. TBI also is called acquired brain injury or just head injury. According to the Centers for Disease Control and Prevention, falls are the leading cause of TBI in adults ages 75 years and older. Motor vehicle accidents are the leading cause in people under 75. In addition, many people get head injuries participating in sports or recreation, from colliding with a moving or stationary object such as a ball or another person, or from an explosion as seen in military combat.

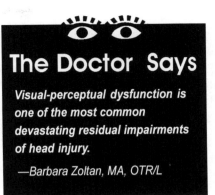

The Doctor Says

Visual-perceptual dysfunction is one of the most common devastating residual impairments of head injury.

—Barbara Zoltan, MA, OTR/L

TBI may rupture blood vessels in the brain or bruise brain tissue. Closed head injuries frequently cause damage right where the head hit. These injuries can affect other areas of the brain as well because the brain has moved back and forth against the inside of the skull from the impact.

Signs of brain damage from TBI may not appear until days or weeks following the injury. The person looks fine but begins to act or feel differently. Besides vision problems, there often are problems with hearing, touch, taste, and smell. Thinking, memory, and reasoning may be affected, as well as communication skills and reading and writing abilities. Behavior or mental health can change, with some of the manifestations being depression, anxiety, personality changes, aggression, acting out, and social inappropriateness.

As a result of Katie's automobile accident, we were very concerned about how her head trauma had affected her visual perception and personality. We noticed a lot of frustration, especially in the assimilation and "processing" of information. We could see her frustration turn to anger, and she would shut out information because it was just too much and too hard for her to try to process. Since vision therapy, the change in Katie is incredible. After vision therapy, Katie is better than ever in her response time, and her ability to assimilate information, and she is back to picking up books and wanting to read.

—Mom

I am able to read again. This is such a pleasure that I used to enjoy before my stroke. I am also able to drive at night without fear of having an accident, and my balance and stamina have gotten so much better as a result of completing vision therapy. I feel so much more independent and can park the car again without hitting anything.

—Connie

Stroke

A stroke happens either when a blood vessel supplying your brain is suddenly blocked or when a blood vessel in the brain bursts. Strokes also are called cerebrovascular accidents (CVA) or "brain attacks." During a stroke, brain cells die when they no longer receive oxygen and nutrients from the blood, or there is sudden bleeding into or around the brain. As with a head injury, part of the brain is damaged during a stroke.

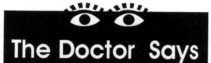

The Doctor Says

Following brain injury, the eyes have a tendency to drift outwards or inwards causing eyestrain, double vision, muscle spasm and excessive peripheral visual stimulation, which in turn can trigger dizziness and balance problems. Treatment is with lenses, prisms and vision therapy.

—Dr. Vincent Vicci
   Neuro-Optometrist
   Westfield, NJ

Unfortunately, many stroke survivors have visual problems following their strokes. Good vision requires the brain and eyes to work together, and the two eyes to work with each other. Depending on the scope of the brain damage, the vision problems can be partial or complete loss of sight and/or vision. Double vision, dizziness, or balance problems are common. Stroke survivors also may experience blurred vision, confusion, or difficulty performing visual activities, and eyestrain. For stroke survivors with vision problems, it is harder to go back to work or even perform simple household tasks. For more information, go to: www.visionhelp.com and www.nora.cc.

Other Neurological Disorders

Epilepsy

Epilepsy often impairs the visual system. Epilepsy is a brain disorder in which clusters of nerve cells or neurons in the brain sometimes signal abnormally. This may affect a person's consciousness, bodily movements, or sensations for a short time.

People with epilepsy can have trouble effectively using both eyes together and interpreting what they see, which diminishes their motor skills, alertness, and attention. Children with epilepsy may not work up to expectations. They may have perfect 20/20 vision, or wear prescribed eyeglasses, but when they read, they lose their place and have to reread the material. They are unable to recall what they have read. They can't follow directions and therefore frequently fail tests. The extra effort they have to expend to read creates even more stress on their already fragile visual systems. They may not be aiming their eyes directly onto the words they are reading and actually may be looking past the page.

Vision problems in people with epilepsy are often subtle and frequently unrecognizable. For both children and adults, neuro-optometric rehabilitation can greatly improve their daily living skills and their ability to meet future challenges.

Cerebral Palsy

Cerebral palsy (CP) is actually a group of chronic disorders that impair one's control of movement. The causes are thought to be incorrect cell development early in pregnancy or damage to a baby's brain cells just after birth, caused by bleeding in the brain, seizures, or breathing and circulation problems. Early signs of CP usually appear before 3 years of age. Infants with CP are

---

The Doctor Says

Doctors and therapists specializing in children and adults with acquired brain injury are becoming more aware and sophisticated regarding the role vision plays in the maintenance of spatial orientation and balance. They are increasingly calling on optometrists to become active members of the rehabilitation process.

—Irwin Suchoff, OD, DOS
Editor of *Visual and Vestibular Consequences of Acquired Brain Injury*

frequently slow to reach developmental milestones such as learning to roll over, sit, crawl, smile, or walk. Symptoms of CP include difficulty writing, using scissors (or other fine motor tasks), difficulty maintaining balance or walking, and displaying involuntary movements. The symptoms differ from person to person and may change over time.

Dr. Appelbaum Talks About His Patient Lily:

Lily was a stroke patient who was first introduced to me while I was seeing patients at the Maryland Adventist Rehabilitation Hospital. She was brought over to me in a wheelchair and wearing a patch over her left eye. She had dizziness and double vision as a result of a stroke, as well as diabetes, hypertension, and high cholesterol. She was receiving daily occupational, speech, and physical therapy at the hospital, with limited progress. Lily was unable to read newspapers, books, or the computer screen. She had had to stop drawing, painting, driving a car, doing ordinary household duties, and taking care of herself, and was unable to walk without feeling as if she were going to fall.

After 2 months of vision therapy in my office, Lily's double vision, dizziness, posture, and gait had improved so much that she was discharged from the rehabilitation hospital and reported that her balance and walking were "much more manageable." After 3 months of vision therapy, she could read newspapers and books, and use the computer for 30 to 40 minutes without eyestrain or discomfort. Lily's drawing improved, and she resumed her beloved hobby of painting. By the fourth month of vision therapy, the double vision was gone and the formerly constant dizziness appeared only once or twice a week. In the vision therapy room, Lily commented: "My disposition has dramatically improved, and I am finally now optimistic about my future."

Her three-dimensional vision appeared for the first time since the stroke— around the fifth month of vision therapy—and Lily reported that the glasses she used all the time were now only needed for reading. "The outdoors and reading are far more pleasurable now. I can walk without feeling like I'm going to fall!"

Two years later, Lily exclaimed: "What a difference 2 years make! I went from not being able to see the Winter Olympics to looking forward to the trials and competition this year. I went from double vision and blurred vision, to what appears to be full correction of my vision problem! My improvement was accompanied by a return of my ability to read fine print, draw and paint, and enjoy video and other games. By the way, I find that many of the new slot machines with a lot of action give my eyes a good workout!"

No standard therapy works for all patients with CP. Drugs can be used to control seizures and muscle spasms. Special braces can compensate for muscle imbalance. Surgery, mechanical aids to help overcome impairments, counseling for emotional and psychological needs, and vision, physical, occupational, speech, and behavioral therapy may be employed. Many people with CP have eyes that are not straight or eyes that may drift only part of the time. Vision therapy often helps with cosmetically noticeable eye-muscle coordination problems. Also, when the eyes look straight, they may still be treatable eye-muscle coordination problems affecting coordination or causing words in print to blur and run together. Some studies note as many as 90 percent of children with CP having trouble keeping the print clear when reading.

If a child or adult with CP is not performing at potential, a vision therapy evaluation needs to be done. Many children and adults with mild CP show tremendous gains in performance after vision therapy.

Multiple Sclerosis

Multiple sclerosis (MS) is a disease of the central nervous system whose effects range from relatively benign to disabling conditions. The disease disrupts communication between the brain and other parts of the body when the body— through its immune system—attacks its own tissues, specifically the insulating covering of nerve cells called myelin. The first symptoms of MS usually appear between the ages of 20 and 40 and include blurred or double vision, red-green color distortion, or blindness in one eye. Most MS patients have muscle weakness in their arms and legs and difficulty with coordination and balance. Half of all people with MS experience cognitive impairments such as difficulties with concentration, attention, memory, and poor judgment, but such symptoms are usually mild and are frequently overlooked. There is as yet no cure for MS.

Vision problems in people with MS can be obvious like double vision, or subtle and frequently unrecognizable. For patients with MS, neuro-optometric rehabilitation and vision therapy can oftentimes greatly improve the quality of their lives.

Vision-Related Symptoms

Many neuro-optometrists group several of the vision-related symptoms associated with head trauma into two general categories: *post-trauma vision syndrome* and *visual midline shift syndrome*. The two syndromes have some of the same symptoms.

Post-Trauma Vision Syndrome

Neuro-optometrists have long recognized visual problems and symptoms associated with head trauma that affect the functional visual system. They call this collection of problems and symptoms post-trauma vision syndrome (PTVS). Head injuries can cause eye alignment imbalances and other difficulties because the visual system is not functioning properly. For example, one eye might turn outward, or it might be hard to get both eyes to work together. Here are some common PTVS symptoms:

- Double vision (diplopia)
- Blurred near vision
- Print seems to move
- Eyestrain (asthenopia)
- Headaches
- Sensitivity to light (photophobia)
- Headaches
- Dizziness, vertigo, balance problems
- Nausea
- Attention or concentration difficulties
- Staring behavior (low blink rate) that causes dry eyes
- Spatial disorientation
- Loses place when reading
- Difficulty finding the beginning of the next line when reading
- Comprehension problems when reading
- Visual memory problems
- Pulling away from objects when they are brought close

The Doctor Says

The majority of people who recover from a traumatic brain injury will have binocular function difficulties in the form of strabismus, phoria, oculomotor dysfunction, convergence, and accommodative abnormalities.

—William Padula, OD

In the past, these symptoms were diagnosed as individual eye problems or eye muscle imbalances. But they are all part of the larger visual system—the relationship of sensory-motor functions controlled and organized in the brain.

Additionally, depending on the extent of the injury, there often are deficits in many areas of visual information-processing abilities. Problems with visual processing may contribute to and or exacerbate symptoms of eyestrain, fatigue, headaches, difficulties with balance and posture, depth perception, memory loss, and excessively slow visual-motor performance affecting handwriting. PTVS can be treated effectively through neuro-optometric rehabilitation. The treatment may include prescribing different lenses in conjunction with therapeutic lenses and prisms, and using other neuro-optometric rehabilitative approaches, including vision therapy.

The Doctor Says

The ultimate purpose of the visual process is to arrive at an appropriate motor and/or cognitive response. There is an extremely high incidence (greater than 50 percent) of visual and visual-cognitive disorders in neurologically impaired patients (traumatic brain injury, cerebral vascular accidents, multiple sclerosis etc.)

—Rosalind Gianutsos, PhD

Visual Midline Shift Syndrome

After people have had a stroke or TBI, vision disorders can occur that cause them to misperceive their position in their own midline. This is known as vision midline shift syndrome (VMSS) and occurs in people with other neurological disabilities as well.[1] The visual perception of the world seems compressed in one portion and expanded in another. The world therefore appears slanted, or tipped, and walls may appear bowed and distorted, which causes patients to lean to one side, or forward, or backward. They have poor balance or posture and often lean back on their heels or lean forward or to one side when walking, standing, or seated in a wheelchair. This often occurs if they have experienced paralysis on one side. Their shifted concept of their

---

[1]Padula, W. 1996. Post-trauma vision syndrome and visual midline shift syndrome. *Neurorehabilitation* 6: 165–171.

visual midline actually reinforces their paralysis. Other symptoms of VMSS include—

- Consistently staying to one side of a hallway or room
- Bumping into objects when walking
- Blurred vision

Dr. Appelbaum Talks About His Patient John:

John was a 60-year-old truck driver who had the good fortune of having a daughter who was a physical therapist. After John had a stroke, he was left with homonymous hemianopsia (visual field loss), strabismus (an eye-teaming problem), and amblyopia (lazy eye). John had major problems keeping his attention centered on reading, could not judge distances accurately, frequently tilted his head, closed or covered one eye when reading, and avoided reading newspapers and books and using the computer. He was confined to a wheelchair because of his poor balance, gait, and posture. John really could not see very well on his left side and, to compensate, had to turn his head "all the way to the left and then slowly to the right." John was suffering from both post-trauma vision syndrome and visual midline shift syndrome.

Before the stroke, he had been left-handed and now he had to be right-handed. Someone now always had to be with him when he went out. His wife now did all the driving and handled the finances. It was very hard for John to enjoy his grandchildren, attend meetings, go boating, or travel—things he used to love to do.

He was not making the kind of progress in occupational, speech, and physical therapy that his daughter expected, so she took him to Johns Hopkins Wilmer Eye Clinic in Baltimore for a thorough evaluation. John saw a team of eye doctors, neurologists, and therapists, but still made very slow progress. Then John was assigned to a new occupational therapist who had recently attended one of my vision therapy workshops. The new therapist insisted that John be evaluated for vision therapy and referred him to me.

After 8 weeks of vision therapy in my office, all of John's therapists, his wife, and he himself noted a significant increase in vision on his (weak) left side, better balance, better walking, and much more reading. A significant reduction of the visual field loss was measured on a computerized Humphrey Visual Field Test. As of this writing, John had had 3 months of vision therapy, and was able to get out of his wheelchair and walk nonstop for up to a half-hour, holding on to a crutch or his wife's hand—all things he had been unable to do during the 2 years after his stroke.

- Sensitivity to light
- Reading difficulties (words appear to move)
- Comprehension difficulty
- Attention and concentration difficulty
- Memory difficulty
- Double vision
- Aching eyes
- Headaches with visual tasks
- Loss of visual field
- Dizziness or nausea, vertigo, balance problems
- Spatial disorientation

Children or adults who have had a stroke, traumatic brain injury, or other neurological insult, often experience a somatic and visual shift in their concept of midline. Objects right in front of them may appear to the right, left, up, or down. When the visual midline shifts, it causes the person to unconsciously think that the body center is shifted in the direction of the visual midline. In turn, the person tends to lean toward the midline shift. This can cause problems with balance, center of gravity, weight bearing, transfer, or walking.

However, when specially designed therapeutic lenses called yoked prisms are prescribed, the patient's midline can be shifted to a more centered position. This frequently enables the patient to begin bearing weight on the paralyzed side.

How Can Vision Therapy Help?

As soon as possible after a head injury or stroke, patients should have a complete eye exam by an eye doctor who specializes in vision therapy to find out if their eyes are healthy and working properly. Neuro-optometrists are important members of the patient's rehabilitation team. They can diagnose specific problems and recommend a treatment plan.

Different types of vision therapy are available to retrain, strengthen, or sharpen vision following head injury or stroke, as well as in people with neurological disabilities. Treatment can range from using computer-like devices to therapeutic lenses, prisms, office, and home procedures. The goal of the therapy is to train healthy parts of the brain to perform the work of the part of the brain that has been damaged. According to research, neither the age of the patient nor when the injury occurred makes a big difference in whether the patient can benefit from vision therapy.

Yoked Prisms

Yoked prisms are therapeutic lenses used in vision therapy. A prism is a wedge of glass or plastic that has a thick end and a thin end. When the thick ends of the prism are positioned in the same direction for each eye, for example, to the right or to the left for both eyes, they are called yoked prisms. Yoked prisms alter a patient's perception of visual space and increase the patient's ability to transfer his or her weight to achieve better posture and balance. These therapeutic prism lenses are not compensatory in nature and are usually prescribed for short periods of time each day, in conjunction with physical and/or occupational therapy.

The initially prescribed power and direction of the yoked prism is only a starting point, and a higher or lower powered prism may be needed, depending on the patient's response to the prism and on the level and intensity of therapy. Frequently, the direction of the yoked prism needs to be changed as therapy progresses. In many cases, the full potential of physical and/or occupational therapy can be reached more quickly when yoked prisms are used. Neuro-optometrically prescribed yoked prisms have been used effectively for many years at neuro-optometric rehabilitation programs in hospitals and rehabilitation centers throughout the United States.

Yoked prism glasses are used therapeutically to alter the visual midline concept of a person who has suffered a neuro-motor imbalance as a result of a stroke, TBI, or a physical disability such as MS or CP. They help shift the visual midline to a more centered position. As mentioned earlier, yoked prism glasses increase the person's ability to transfer weight over to the affected side.

Physical and occupational therapy rehabilitation for TBI, stroke, or other neurological disorders often plateaus and reaches a limit if the visual midline shift has not been addressed with yoked prisms, therapeutic lenses, and vision

My son did vision therapy because he had frequent bad headaches and double vision at least in part from his eyes not tracking together. He was in a car accident, which caused this problem. He was unable to read more than a few minutes at a time; his concentration was bad; his pleasure in reading was very low. His body coordination was poor. He became clumsy when he used to be just the opposite. We had already gone to a psychologist, neurologist, and psychiatrist. They were only of minimal assistance and mainly just gave him meds for the pain. The doctor doing the vision therapy changed his eyeglass prescription and also advised his occupational and physical therapists on procedures. Since vision therapy, my son now has almost no headaches and seldom experiences double vision anymore, instead of being in almost constant pain. He can now concentrate again on his schoolwork. He reads for pleasure again for many hours, taking small breaks to rest his eyes. His coordination is once again very good.

—Mom

therapy. These treatments often enhance the effect of physical and occupational therapy. Prescription of yoked prisms may include low amounts of prism incorporated in the person's glasses and a second higher amount of yoked prism for short-term use in conjunction with occupational or physical therapy. Yoked prisms also can improve muscle tone as well as imbalances in facial muscles, posture, and orientation.

People who have a neurological vision problem often will mention their symptoms to their physician and rehabilitative therapists, who may recommend a routine eye exam rather than a neuro-optometric exam. The result is that the eye doctor finds that the visual acuity and the health of the eyes are normal and that "the patient's problems are not related to the eyes." In addition, if there are balance disorders, persons will be referred for physical and occupational therapy or vestibular evaluation and treatment. In many cases, if the underlying visual-processing problem is not determined and treated, there will be limited progress. A neuro-optometric rehabilitation treatment plan improves the specific acquired visual deficits that are identified during the neuro-optometric evaluation.

Neuro-optometric rehabilitation involves a treatment regimen incorporating lenses, prisms, low-vision aids, and vision therapy activities designed to relieve vision symptoms and increase vision efficiency. This in turn can help support many other activities of daily living. Neuro-optometric rehabilitation retrains the brain, eye muscles, and body. The following sections show how vision therapy can rehabilitate some of the common symptoms found in people who have had TBI, a stroke, or other neurological disorders.

Double Vision

Double vision occurs when we perceive two images from a single object. The images can be horizontal, vertical, or diagonal. Double vision happens when the two eyes are not correctly aligned while aiming at an object and instead are aimed at different objects. Therefore, the eyes send two different images to the brain, and the brain accepts and uses the two unmatched images simultaneously. Double vision causes confusion and disorientation. People with double vision are often given an eye patch, which does resolve the problem but also reduces their field of vision, interferes with normal visual judgments in space, and makes movement in space difficult and hazardous. Double vision can often be eliminated without an eye patch through therapeutic lenses, prisms, and vision therapy.

Reading Difficulty

Difficulty in reading may be caused by visual problems such as blurred or double vision, jerky eye movements, and visual field loss, making it difficult to keep one's place on a page. Relief can usually be obtained with appropriate reading glasses, prisms, and vision therapy, depending on the specific case. Moving a ruler down the page, line by line, can make it easier to keep one's place when the problem is jerky eye movements or visual field loss. Some patients find it easier to read and keep their place by using a typoscope, which is a sheet of black cardboard or plastic with a cutout the size of a line of print. The typoscope isolates the line that is being read. Patients simply move the typoscope across each line of print and then down to the next line.

Visual Field Loss

The normal human visual field extends to approximately 60 degrees nasally (toward the nose, or inward) in each eye, to 100 degrees temporally (away from the nose, or outwards), and approximately 60 degrees above and 75 below the horizontal meridian. Head injury often causes severe impairments to the field of vision. Of the many possible visual field impairments, the two most common are called *hemianopsia* and *unilateral neglect*.

In hemianopsia, up to half of the visual field is lost, on either one's left or right side. People with the condition see nothing to the left or to the right of the object they are looking at. They bump into walls and doorways, fail to see objects and people in the affected field, knock over cups and glasses, and commit other mishaps. Hemianopsia makes driving extremely hazardous.

Unilateral neglect is a condition caused by injury usually to the brain's parietal lobe. The left visual field is more commonly affected. People with unilateral neglect, like those with hemianopsia, do not see objects on one side. Therefore, they too frequently bump into walls, doorways, and objects, and fail to see people and objects on the affected side. In addition, they ignore one side of their own body. They do not dress that side, or shave or apply makeup to that side of the face. They may even fail to see one side of various objects, whether the objects are located in the left or the right visual field. When asked to draw a daisy or a clock, they may place all the petals on the right side of the daisy, or cram all 12 numbers of the clock dial onto the right side.

Much can be done to help people who suffer from hemianopsia and unilateral neglect. Although the visual field loss is caused by nerve damage, often the prescription of yoked prism lenses and neuro-optometric therapy will help patients identify objects in the affected field and therefore react and process at a more functional level. Yoked prisms and mirror devices are often helpful. Various exercises are designed to increase awareness, sensitivity, and use of the vision remaining in the affected field. Recent research released at the 2007 International Stroke Conference in San Francisco indicated that more than 75 percent of patients with stroke and traumatic brain injury reported visual field improvements from vision rehabilitation intervention, confirming previous research. Vision therapy, like occupational, physical, and speech therapy, is currently thought to help the brain to adapt, based on the concept of neuroplasticity, and form new connections to compensate for injury.

Low Vision

Some people with acquired brain injury have a normal field of vision but cannot read ordinary print or watch television because they cannot see clearly and sharply even with conventional glasses. They have reduced visual acuity, or low vision. Neuro-optometric rehabilitation can help them handle daily activities and maintain independence. Low-vision aids include sophisticated telescopic lenses for distance vision, magnifying lenses, and complex microscopic and electronic magnifiers for reading and other fine tasks.

Dry Eye

If the nerves or muscles of the eyelids are affected by stroke or head injury, the lids may not close fully on each blink or during sleep, causing the gritty, burning secretion associated with dry eye. Dry-eye symptoms can be relieved by patients applying carefully selected lubricating drops and ointments, and by drinking at least eight, 8-ounce glasses of water per day. In severe cases, collagen plugs inserted into their tear ducts frequently work to increase lubrication of the eyes and eliminate discomfort.

Visual-Perceptual-Motor and Information-Processing Deficits

People with acquired brain injury frequently experience unstable orientation in space, so that objects, and even the walls and floor, seem to move and shift about. They also have difficulty with object localization and visual judgments in space, inability to sustain visual attention, and poor visual memory. These functions can often be improved through the use of prisms that restore their ability to orient themselves in space, as well as rehabilitative vision therapy to improve their visual perceptual, spatial, and information-processing functions. Behavioral observations during therapy sessions or medical examinations, in-depth interviews, and screenings provide information about potential visual dysfunctions.

Dr. Appelbaum Talks About His Patient Peter:

Peter was a high school English teacher. As it turned out, my daughter was assigned to his English class at the beginning of her senior year. At dinner after her first day of classes, she announced that she had a substitute teacher for English because her teacher was sick. The next day, my first patient was none other than Peter, who had recently had a car accident and suffered a brain injury. Peter had been referred to me by his occupational and physical therapists at the rehabilitation hospital. He was a Shakespearean scholar who loved to read but could not read now for more than a few minutes without feeling sleepy. This problem was caused by convergence (eye teaming) and accommodative (focusing) deficits that caused blurring, double vision, jerky eye movements, and visual field loss, which made it difficult for him to keep his place on a page.

Peter needed appropriate reading glasses, prisms, and vision therapy. Moving a ruler down the page line by line, he found it easier to temporarily keep his place on the page. I then had him read with a typoscope, a sheet of black cardboard or plastic with a cutout the size of a line of print that isolated the line that was being read. The typoscope made it easier to keep his place and to focus. Peter simply moved the typoscope across each line of print, and then down to the next line. Luckily, Peter was identified and referred directly from the rehabilitation hospital to me and therefore was reading again in a few months. After Peter's third month of vision therapy, my daughter finally met her English teacher, because he could read well enough to go back to work.

Sports and Vision Therapy

Do you play soccer, tennis, basketball, baseball, or any other game involving moving balls and other players? Are you satisfied with your performance? If you are not, have you ever asked yourself what the problem could be?

In tennis or golf, do you frequently hit the ball on the edge of the racquet or club, or miss it completely? In basketball or baseball, can you shoot baskets accurately, or catch a fly ball in center field? Have you wondered why your child cannot even come close to scoring a goal on the soccer field?

The Doctor Says

Coaches tell us to keep our eyes on the ball but fail to provide the drills and techniques for improving this skill.

—Dr. Bryce Appelbaum

It is not enough to just say "Keep your eye on the ball." As we have repeatedly emphasized, vision is much more than being able to see clearly. Nothing really happens in sports until the eyes tell the hands and body what to do. If your eyes do not instruct your hands and body what to do, performance on the playing field, court, or course suffers! Strong, adequately developed visual skills and abilities are critical to sports success.

The Doctor Says

Outstanding sports performance is very much related to outstanding visual skills. Studies show that approximately 80 percent of perceptual input in sports is visual.

—Dr. Bryce Appelbaum

If you or your child cannot seem to reach full potential, no matter how hard you have practiced or how many years you have put into it, it may be time to give your visual system a workout. You have probably been given advice on nutrition, weight training, rest, stretching, psychology, and so on, but almost nothing on improving your vision. Vision therapy can improve your brain's ability to process visual information and your body's ability to respond to it.

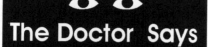

The Doctor Says

Inadequately developed visual skills make it difficult but not impossible to play ball sports. Inconsistent performance, decreasing performance as the pressure increases, or skilled performance only when the body is stationary or in balance, and not when moving or out of balance are frequently vision problems causing sports problems.

—Dr. Bryce Appelbaum

Professional sports organizations know this. They are increasingly using sports vision therapy in their training regimens. The National Basketball Association, the PGA Tour, the U.S. Olympic bobsled and luge teams, Nascar racers, skeet shooters, trap shooters, minor- and major-league baseball and football players and teams all have integrated vision therapy into their training programs.

The key to success in sports, whether you play on the high school team or the U.S. Olympic team, is having both natural athletic abilities, training, AND great visual skills and abilities. Studies have shown that superior visual skills correlate with superior performance, and poor visual skills impede your performance. The body's timing is affected by errors in visual judgment that result in mistakes on the playing field, court, or course.

Approximately 80 percent of the cues for playing most sports are sensed through vision. Therefore, your visual skills and abilities must be reliable under pressure, whether you are playing a weekly game of tennis or trying to become a professional tennis player. As you know, 20/20 eyesight means only that you can see a small object clearly at a distance. Having good eyesight is not enough. Your visual system must be able to gather many kinds of information: for example, where the ball is located in space, how fast it is traveling, where you are located in relationship to the ball, where you need to be, and where the ball needs to go. It is only through adequately developed visual processing that the weekend or professional athlete gathers this information.

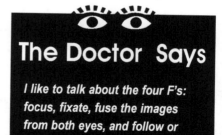

The Doctor Says

I like to talk about the four F's: focus, fixate, fuse the images from both eyes, and follow or track an image through space.

—Dr. Sue E. Lowe

Super Bowl Receiver Credits Vision Therapy

One player in the 2009 Super Bowl was given a major advantage over others while still a child. The 25 year-old wide receiver for the Arizona Cardinals, Larry Fitzgerald, has a grandfather and aunt who are Optometrists specializing in Vision Therapy in Chicago. These Optometrists first worked with Larry as a child to improve his visual attention and academic performance. Larry was an exuberant child, always on the go. The vision therapy procedures he worked on during summers with his optometric family in Chicago helped him academically.

The Doctor Says

Optimal sports visual performance is making the appropriate response in the shortest period of time based on the least amount of information, with the least amount of effort, in or out of balance and for extended periods of time.

—Gary Etting, OD, FCOVD

When Larry turned 12, his grandfather recognized his athletic gifts and adapted many of the vision therapy procedures to develop high level eye-hand coordination. For example, to improve Larry's visual control, spatial judgment and rhythm, Dr. Johnson would hang a painted ball from the ceiling and have him try to hit the colored dots on the ball with the matching colored stripes on a rolling pin.

All of the doctors in the VisionHelp.com network utilize this procedure, known as the Marsden Ball, to assist patients of all ages develop to their full visual potential.

To read more about this amazing wide receiver and the power of Optometric Vision Therapy in helping mold him not only as a gifted athlete, but as a gifted individual, go to www.VisionHelp.com/sports3.htm

What Vision Skills Are Important for Sports?

Your vision is composed of many interrelated skills that can affect how well you play your sport. Sports vision skills are about coordinating your eyes, brain, hands, feet, and body. These skills include all of those we have discussed earlier that are needed for reading and classroom work, with additional emphasis on visual stamina, speed, agility, and coordination.

From .206 to .282!

Greg Vaughn, the former San Diego Padres left-fielder, was voted to the All-Star team in 1998 and led the Padres into the playoffs with a .282 batting average. He attributed much of his success that year to vision therapy, along with good coaching and more playing time. San Diego Union sports columnist Tom Cushman called it "the most astonishing turnaround I've witnessed in 30-plus years of covering major-league baseball." Vaughn worked with San Diego behavioral optometrist Dr. Carl Hillier and his staff of vision therapists. In spite of Vaughn's good visual skills, Dr. Hillier found high-level visual inefficiencies that were limiting Vaughn's ability to perform to his full potential. Vaughn began a program of vision therapy designed to enhance the speed and accuracy of his visual motor response to visual stimuli. After several sessions, Vaughn reported that "a 95 mph fast ball looks like it's coming in at 88 mph!" Vaughn's improvement resulted in the referral of several other Padre players, as well as those from other teams to Dr. Hillier, to begin vision therapy programs. He was also the catalyst for several national media articles, as well as an outstanding ESPN interview that highlighted the important relationship between vision and hitting. Vaughn has stated, "The whole concept for going to vision therapy is to be able to pick up and recognize objects and get the information from my eyes to my brain—taking advantage of opportunities you have to make yourself better."

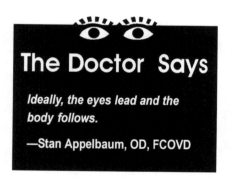

The Doctor Says

Ideally, the eyes lead and the body follows.

—Stan Appelbaum, OD, FCOVD

Good eyesight (at least 20/20) is a prerequisite. Poor eyesight undermines all the other visual skills and abilities and should be corrected if necessary with contact lenses, eyeglasses, laser surgery, or alternatively through a combination of Orthokeratology (Ortho-K—defined in the next section), stress-relieving lenses, and vision therapy.

The American Optometric Association lists nine vision skills important for success at sports:

- *Dynamic visual acuity*—Your ability to see objects clearly while you, the ball, or both at the same time, are moving. You are able to shift where you are looking from far to near.

- *Visual concentration*—Helps you screen out distractions and stay focused on the ball or the target.

- *Eye tracking*—Your eyes can follow moving objects efficiently. This helps you maintain balance and react to a situation quickly.
- *Eye-hand-body coordination*—How your hands, feet, and body respond to the things you see.
- *Visual memory*—Your ability to remember a fast-moving, complex picture of people and things. This enables you to learn from previous experience and quickly get where you need to be.

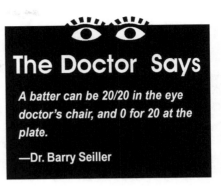

The Doctor Says

A batter can be 20/20 in the eye doctor's chair, and 0 for 20 at the plate.

—Dr. Barry Seiller

- *Visualization*—Your ability to imagine yourself by seeing a mental movie of yourself performing well while at the same time your eyes are seeing and concentrating on something else, usually the ball. Visualization can be used as a warm-up and practice before competition.

- *Peripheral vision*—Seeing things out of the side of each eye without having to turn your head. After all, much of what happens in sports is not directly in front of you.
- *Visual reaction time*—The speed with which your brain interprets and reacts to the layout of the field and/or your opponent's action.
- *Depth perception*—Being able to quickly and accurately judge the distance between yourself, the ball, your opponents, teammates, boundary lines, and other objects.

How Does Vision Therapy Help?

Different sports have different visual demands. Amateur and professional athletes need different approaches. An optometrist with expertise in sports vision can assess your unique visual system and perform a basic eye exam. To avoid having to wear contacts or eyeglasses, some people consider laser surgery to first correct their eyesight. By gently and safely reshaping the cornea (front surface of the eye) with custom contact lenses, Orthokeratology (Ortho-K or corneal refractive therapy) plus stress-reducing lenses and vision therapy are an alternative to laser surgery. For more information on Ortho-K, go to www.visionhelp.com.

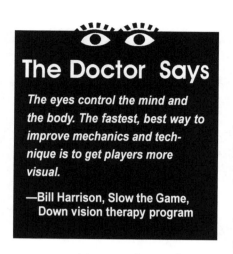

The Doctor Says

The eyes control the mind and the body. The fastest, best way to improve mechanics and technique is to get players more visual.

—Bill Harrison, Slow the Game, Down vision therapy program

After the eye exam, the doctor assesses your visual skills to determine, for example, whether one of your eyes is dominant and if your eyes are working effectively together. You will be asked to look at images with each eye, first separately and then together. Your ability to quickly recognize and respond to an image will be observed, as well as how well you track an object moving in space. Your depth perception will also be assessed.

Your eye-hand coordination, visual reaction time, peripheral awareness, eye teaming, focusing, tracking, and visualization skills are some of the abilities the doctor can evaluate, train, and enhance.

Adults and children who seek help from optometrists often have serious learning problems or other disabilities, all of which may be barriers to good sports performance as well. Time and time again, patients who have undergone vision therapy to alleviate the visual symptoms that worsen attention deficit hyperactivity disorder, autism, and other disabilities, report joyfully that they can finally participate in their chosen sports activities.

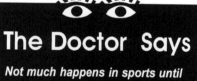

The Doctor Says

Not much happens in sports until your eyes instruct your hands and body as to what to do

—Carole Burns, OD, FCOVD
  Maxsportscenter.com
  Columbus, Ohio

Dr. Appelbaum Talks About His Patient Noah:

Noah had participated in almost every rifle event for several years with the goal of making the 2000 Olympic Games in Australia. He practiced daily and had several coaches work with him to improve the accuracy of his shooting. Then he started to read about the visual skills involved in becoming a competitive Olympic shooter. He learned that vision is important in every sports activity, affecting coordination, concentration, balance, and accuracy. So Noah began vision therapy with me, receiving two treatment sessions per week in the office and practicing daily at home. After a year of treatment, Noah's very good visual skills and abilities became excellent visual skills and abilities, and he ended up making the Olympic Team with outstanding results!

Vision therapy, by training you to more efficiently use your visual system, improves your self-confidence. You are visually and physically connected with the game you are playing and not distracted by irrelevant visual stimuli.

What Are the Current Approaches?

These days, sports vision therapy clinics are using sophisticated approaches to enhance their patients' vision. For example, there are *tinted contact lenses* designed to make the ball stand out. Some lenses filter out specific wavelengths of light to enhance other elements in one's view. Grey-green lenses are designed for sports played in bright sunlight, and amber lenses are for sports like tennis and soccer that require tracking a fast-moving ball.

Computerized vision-training programs have been developed that can be used either in a training facility or at home. The *conditioned ocular enhancement training system* for baseball players shoots out tennis balls inscribed with a red or black number from 1 to 9. The machine is designed to improve the player's concentration on the ball. The hitter stands about 60 feet away and taking his normal batting position, tracks the ball to the plate, trying to read the number and color.

A typical exercise will start shooting the ball at 90 miles per hour (game speed) and increase it to 150 miles per hour. When returned to the original speed, and later during a real game, the ball seems much slower and larger. Players are put through any number of drills to improve their depth perception and ability to track a ball. For example, one drill teaches players to visualize merging two slightly different pictures held up a few inches apart. Players then can more easily learn to read the ball's speed and changes in speed.

What About Laser Surgery and Corneal Refractive Therapy (Orthokeratology)?

Laser surgery is popular among athletes these days as an alternative to eyeglasses and contact lenses. Athletes who play in fields may choose to have laser surgery because of the constant problems with their contact lenses caused by dirt and wind. The surgery reshapes the cornea to correct nearsightedness and farsightedness. It also has been found to reduce glare so that players squint less and can open their eyes wider.

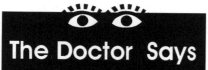

The Doctor Says

Corneal refractive therapy (Ortho-K) allows athletes to be contact lens free and glasses free (without eye surgery) when around dirt, dust, or wind.

—Dr. Carole Burns

Orthokeratology (Ortho-K or corneal refractive therapy) involves wearing special contact lenses, usually only at night, that reshape the cornea. This method can be used as an effective nonsurgical alternative to laser surgery, for correcting near- and farsightedness. A number of FDA-approved lenses are now available. The contact lenses reshape the cornea through gentle compression by causing a very small movement of cells that cover the surface of the cornea.

Dr. Appelbaum Talks About His Patient Jason:

Just recently, Jason finally became part of a major-league baseball team. In college, he had been described as the cornerstone of his team. He was defensively and offensively outstanding. He could steal bases. He was described as the total package. Jason really could swing the bat with great arm strength. The problem was he had difficulty picking up the ball and seeing the ball out of the pitcher's hand. The issue was depth perception and problems with visual reaction time. His batting average was a respectable .272, but he wanted to get it much higher. Jason came to see me with the goal of reaching his "full potential as an athlete and as a person." Visual performance testing indicated that Jason often had tired eyes after reading, problems with being 100 percent focused during games and with judging the strike zone, difficulty with being "in the zone" while playing ball and with consistently seeing the ball out of the pitcher's hand and tracking it to the plate. Also, he frequently felt "eyestrain" at game time.

After 3 months of vision therapy at my office, Jason had a vast improvement. He felt he was able to track the baseball much better, and his visual reaction time had dramatically increased. His batting average jumped to .350. Jason was astonished to also see a huge improvement in his reading comprehension and was now reading a book a week, on average, for the first time in his life. He told me he had been playing ping pong with a childhood friend for years and finally was consistently winning. His friend was unaware of Jason's vision therapy and wanted to know what vitamins Jason was on, so he could also get some!

Jason's progress evaluation showed significant reduction of his binocular instability, much improved convergence, less oculomotor suppression, increased focus stamina, and a much better balance between his two eyes even though Jason had better than 20/20 eyesight in both eyes before beginning vision therapy. Jason's "eyesight" had been fine, but it was his "vision" that needed to be improved.

Vision Therapy in Action

By now you must be curious about the nuts and bolts of vision therapy. What exactly would you have to do in a vision therapy program? How difficult would it be?

We would be misleading you if we were to claim vision therapy is a breeze. It is not. It is hard work—daily focused practice and regular visits to the vision therapist, usually for months. Stress must be exerted on your mind/body system so that you can stretch your capacity, learn new skills, and raise your level of performance. Causing new circuits and connections to form in the brain takes time and effort.

A vision therapy program can be compared in some ways to training programs designed to achieve proficiency in music, football, or the martial arts. Or, to think of it a little differently, vision therapy is similar to physical therapy or rehabilitation after a stroke. All of these involve discipline and determination on the part of the trainee, but they also require supervision—by a teacher, a coach, or therapist. Even though you must force yourself and teach yourself, you cannot be fully effective without professional supervision.

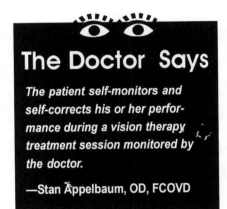

The Doctor Says

The patient self-monitors and self-corrects his or her performance during a vision therapy treatment session monitored by the doctor.

—Stan Appelbaum, OD, FCOVD

This applies to vision therapy too. It is not a do-it-yourself program, yet it has a self-monitoring, self-directing, and self-correcting component. It requires a high level of motivation.

The first step must always be a diagnosis of the problem ideally by an optometrist board certified in vision development and vision therapy by the College of Optometric Vision Development (COVD) (www.covd.org). The doctor then designs a training program aimed at reducing or eliminating your particular visual deficiencies and related problems or enhancing your visual skills and abilities. The program will usually contain both supervised office treatment and guided but unsupervised home procedures.

A number of fairly standard vision therapy procedures, balancing activities, and related training techniques—many of them derived from the workshops, seminars, and courses of the COVD and the Optometric Extension Program (www.oepf.org) —are used by most behavioral optometrists. The procedures are designed to achieve better body awareness, better body balance and coordination, greater ability to take in "more space" through the eyes, improvement in your perception of "size constancy," and greater range, smoothness, and flexibility in your eyes' response to visual tasks. Some of these are described later in this chapter. Each doctor prescribes his or her own mix of office and home procedures, specifically tailored to the particular problems and capacities of each patient, but within the parameters of professional guidelines. Procedures with lenses and prisms are almost always performed in the office under close professional supervision. We talk about the special importance of lenses in Chapter 9. A range of training exercises is described in Chapter 10.

The Doctor Says

One of my favorite books on vision therapy, which has been acknowledged by many therapists and doctors as the standard textbook in the field is "Applied Concepts in Vision Therapy *by Leonard Press, OD, FCOVD (www.oep.org/press-acvt).*

—Stan Appelbaum, OD, FCOVD

Some behavioral optometrists see their patients once or twice a week and expect them to do 10 to 30 minutes of training at home each day. The home procedures help the patient practice and perfect what has been learned in the office under the direct supervision of the doctor. Patients who live very far away from their behavioral optometrist see them only once every several weeks, and their training is done mainly at home. Many very young children are given home procedures to do under the supervision of their parents, and see their behavioral optometrist weekly or monthly. Motivated patients can complete the office treatment program in as short a time as 6 to 8 months with one or two office sessions per week. Complicated cases such as after eye muscle surgery with amblyopia (lazy eye) can take much longer.

Goals in Your Vision Therapy Program

Behavioral optometrists sometimes differ from one another on particular training techniques. However, most would agree on the three fundamental purposes of the therapy:

- To move you away from your present visual problems causing inefficient performance
- To get your body/mind system moving toward improved integration
- To achieve and sustain a higher quality of visual performance

A training program always starts with a careful assessment followed by establishment of goals for optimum visual performance. The goals are based on a careful analysis of your visual problem, age, energy level, and capacity for undertaking a possibly stressful training program. The analysis looks at whether you have a visual deficiency in urgent need of correction, have only a moderate problem, are about to develop a vision problem and in need of a preventive treatment program, or are seeking primarily to enhance an already excellent performance.

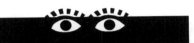

The Doctor Says

Eye Doctors who practice vision therapy are concerned not just with how well people see, but with how well they are able to use their eyes and how comfortably they can sustain concentration and attention.

Henry M. Friedman, OD

Goals help to guide and measure a complicated process. When you are in vision therapy, performing a variety of vision, body-awareness, and balancing improvement techniques over a period of weeks and months, the interactions between your eyes, brain, and the muscular and nervous systems throughout your body are highly complex. Your doctor and therapist can observe changes in visual performance to find clues as to which procedures should be reinforced, which should be curtailed, and whether a given pace of training is appropriate under the circumstances.

An example is the case of Townsend Hoopes, Ann's husband. Here is his story:

Townsend's Story

Townsend's behavioral optometrist, Dr. Appelbaum, made these notations in his initial assessment: "(a) the patient looked fatigued; (b) slumped posture generally, with a leftward tilt to the shoulders and also a head tilt; (c) walked as though the upper part of his body had nothing to do with the lower part; (d) heavy lower body; (e) heavily muscled overall; (f) obviously he was exerting a great deal of energy to handle his body; (g) asked good questions."

Dr. Appelbaum conducted an analytical vision performance examination that revealed "stress-induced type of vision problem, complicated by a vertical phoria causing the right eye to aim higher than the left; unaided acuity (eyesight) at distance is poor enough to cause stress, and so is his corrected acuity at near." It was also indicated that "the patient pours a great deal of energy into seeing at both far and near; measures of reserve energy are low; there is a definite tilt in his visual performance consistent with his body tilt." The basic conclusion was that Townsend was "going all out" to achieve reasonable binocular efficiency.

From this assessment, Dr. Appelbaum developed goals for improved performance: (a) a significant reduction of visual stress at both near point and distance, (b) improved acuity at near point and distance, (c) elimination of the postural slump and the leftward tilt, and (d) more energy.

The doctor first gave Townsend low-plus single-vision reading glasses with a much larger lens area than his current glasses. Townsend had been wearing half-glasses for reading, and a progressive invisible bifocal that restricted the area of visual intake. The mere fact that the new glasses allowed him to cover a wider field made seeing and reading immediately easier.

Dr. Appelbaum then designed a training program aimed primarily at relieving the stress in Townsend's system while moving gradually to strengthen his distance vision. The elements included body awareness and balancing exercises to create a greater "physical looseness" and to improve his "gross balancing ability." Townsend also was instructed to walk and jog several times a week to break down the "artificial barriers" between his upper and lower body and to move him toward a more harmonious visual-postural alignment. In addition, Townsend did simple vision therapy procedures at home to strengthen his ability to shift smoothly from near focus to far focus and vice versa. In Dr. Appelbaum's office, Townsend performed procedures with "doubling prism glasses" and other training lenses, under Dr. Appelbaum's supervision. All of these activities were done at a reasonable pace so as to avoid a "transition" reaction severe enough to take Townsend away from his job for even a few days.

Townsend's initial compliance with the program did not meet the doctor's expectations, but his enthusiasm and diligence improved as progress became evident. Townsend's unaided distance vision improved from 20/60 to 20/40 over 6 months, and the vertical phoria was reduced by 80 percent. His eyestrain was virtually gone, which gave him the sense of enjoying a measurably higher level of energy. Townsend felt he was handling his workload and life in general with greater efficiency, less stress, and more satisfaction. His tennis and golf game dramatically improved.

Inconsistencies and Mismatches?

A primary purpose of vision therapy is to get you to take a hard look at what you see versus what is really there. In a vision therapy program, your doctor tries to show you that there are inconsistencies, or a mismatch, between what you know the real world to be like, versus the way you see it. Most people with vision problems make a conscious effort to believe that the world they see is consistent with the reality they know intellectually. Often, maintaining this sense of consistency requires suspending our judgment—suppressing our subconscious awareness that there are in fact disturbing inconsistencies between what we see and what we know to be the reality.

> **The Doctor Says**
>
> *The mind is very plastic. You can become better at processing visual information at any age.*
>
> —Dr. Sue E. Lowe

In order to help you develop normal binocular vision, the doctor will concentrate on the mismatch between what you see and what really is there. This will help you utilize self-monitoring and self-control to develop the appropriate visual skills and abilities.

For example, a patient may report to the doctor that the wall of the room before him seems to be about 3 feet high, even though he is aware that when he stands up, the ceiling is 2 feet above his head. When the patient is then asked if the ceiling and the floor look perfectly horizontal and do not converge toward each other at any point, and he replies yes, the doctor confronts him with the discrepancy: if the ceiling and floor appear to be horizontal, but the wall looks only 3 feet high, how then does the patient account for the missing 5 feet of space between the 3-foot wall and the 8-foot ceiling? The patient must face up to the truth that the way he sees the world through his eyes is not the world as it really is. These visual-spatial-localization problems are frequently seen in patients with head injury but can also be seen in patients without head injury.

The Doctor Says

Almost any symptom I can create in the exam chair, I can help my patient eliminate in their daily lives with therapeutic lenses and vision therapy.

—Stan Appelbaum, OD, FCOVD

In another example, the vision therapist asks you to try to focus your eyes on a target 10 feet away. You try this and believe you are doing exactly what is asked, but the phoropter (visual testing instrument) shows that your eyes are converging at a distance of 22 inches. Unable to deny this demonstrated inconsistency, you might feel a temporary disorientation, sometimes called "critical empathy." This may be accompanied by nausea or headache. One of Dr. Appelbaum's patients actually fainted during this disorientation. Some patients will say the testing makes them feel "carsick." Motion sickness, carsickness, vertigo, and dizziness are oftentimes vision problems that can be helped with therapeutic lenses and vision therapy.

Your doctor must judge your condition before confronting you with these visual inconsistencies, and the timing can be important. Behavioral optometrists believe it is essential to bring you face to face with your inconsistencies. You then usually achieve a genuine breakthrough—meaning that your visual perceptions thereafter begin to move more in the direction of reality.

There is really no risk when doing vision therapy with a doctor who is board certified (FCOVD). Medications and surgery are generally not used in vision therapy. However, a brief trauma or "transition" may occur when, as a result of vision therapy, your eyes begin seeing in a different way, but before your body has been able to assimilate the change. For example, when you suddenly, for the first time in your life, see the world in the third dimension or achieve a sharper, brighter sense of color, your body/mind system is temporarily out of synch. The reaction may be exhilaration or depression, but there is always a feeling of disorientation. This is what happened to Dr. Susan Barry ("Stereo Sue") when she first experienced binocular vision (discussed in Chapter 5). Oliver Sacks, MD, the famous neurologist, wrote about her experiences on the road to binocular vision in the June 19, 2006 *New Yorker Magazine* article, "Two Eyes Are Better Than ONE... the Blessings of Binocular Vision." Vision therapists know this disorientation is a positive sign, and that a better matching of the visual and body systems will be the result.

Regular physical conditioning, including body-awareness exercises (described in Chapter 10), provides an important safeguard against the temporary discomfort of changes that often take place in the muscles of the neck and upper back (and ultimately throughout the body) following a visual change. Physical conditioning will also cushion the emotional reaction to visual change. Going through vision therapy under the expert guidance of a doctor who is board certified (FCOVD), helps manage these reactions. Where the training is carefully paced and supervised by the doctor, most patients experience only mild and brief disorganization en route to a visual breakthrough.

Poor Timing and Coordination

In addition to the serious inconsistencies and mismatches we have been talking about, there are lesser visual problems that require improvement in coordinating your visual system with your hand and body movements. The problem may be something as obvious as a child's inability to keep her eyes on a moving target. Or, when tracking such a target, she may jerk her head or her whole body in an excessive effort to control a movement that should be smooth and automatic. When she must work hard just at the physical act of seeing, this interferes with her understanding of what she is seeing. Or, think of a teenager learning to drive a stick-shift car: he is so involved with the mechanics of steering and shifting gears that he just does not see what is going on around him.

The problem may be less obvious. It may be a subtle difficulty in timing—being slightly out of step in the coordination between eye and hand. This problem causes a small corrective adjustment after each move, which disturbs the rhythm of body coordination and interferes with your ability to interpret what you are seeing. A child may lose her place while reading; she may reverse letters or words, or fail to recognize subtle changes in the meaning of materials being presented. People with this kind of visual difficulty find it hard to see precise similarities and differences between various elements in a given physical, intellectual, or social situation. Therefore, they might fail to see how certain combinations of elements can be made to fit together in a meaningful way.

Body-Awareness Procedures

Vision therapy procedures to improve body awareness involve a continuous three-step process:

- The visual system receives stimuli.
- The mind processes the stimuli and sends instructions.
- The body responds.

These two office procedures are designed to improve body awareness. In the first, you walk slowly across the room calling out, and simultaneously executing such instructions as "right hand up, right hand down, left foot up, left foot down." The basic idea is: "Say what you do and do what you say." A variation of this exercise, called Angels in the Snow, is performed as you are lying face up on the floor. You call out the instructions in a prescribed sequence and move your arms and legs accordingly—for example, "Right arm and right leg out. Both arms out, both arms in." These movements are performed to the beat of a metronome—one word for each beat, 40 beats per minute.

At first, patients doing these exercises often have trouble matching the spoken instruction with the body response. For example, they will call out "right hand up" while they are in fact lifting the left hand. The doctor or therapist never corrects the patient for a miscall, but repeats the basic instruction. The doctor or therapist insists that patients evaluate their own performance and correct their own mistakes. Intervention would defeat the primary purpose of the exercise, which is to give the patient a firsthand experience in body awareness, synchronization of mind and body, coordination, and control.

Other exercises designed specifically to improve your body awareness, balance, and coordination are known as the Ballet, the Balance Rail, and Bilateral Motor Equivalents. These are described in Chapter 10. All are based on the assumption that humans are self-directing, self-correcting organisms and that vision is the dominant learning process—the central mediator and coordinator in the body/mind system. Poor body awareness can indicate emotional issues, but as the former improves, so does the latter. Some patients even report that improvements in their visual-postural performance and body awareness have improved their golf, tennis, and other sports games.

Yet another procedure is known as "standing awareness," which consists of standing comfortably with both eyes closed for periods of 10 to 30 minutes. This procedure is especially useful when there is mismatch between your visual and body awareness, because it requires you to come to terms with your body posture. Often we do not have an accurate feel for the contours of our body and the space it occupies. For example, we are not aware that our back is "dented in" or that our neck is thrust forward; we do not sense that our hips or our head are slightly twisted, or that we are carrying more weight on one leg than on the other. While the doctor—or anyone else looking closely— can see these deficiencies, it is difficult to explain them persuasively to the patient. The value of standing awareness is that it encourages us to discover these deficiencies for ourselves.

A second purpose of the standing-awareness procedure is to develop a sense of body balance without the help or hindrance of visual reference points. The true centers of balance are the middle of your pelvic area and the middle of your chest. Standing awareness teaches you to concentrate on these central points as you stand with both eyes closed. Concentrating on your "center" while doing the standing-awareness exercise will gradually help you achieve a more natural and balanced posture.

The standing-awareness procedure must be approached with caution and good judgment, and must always be conducted under professional supervision because it can produce in some patients an emotional reaction. As you do the exercise, you attempt to put your mind in neutral and to "think" through your body alone. You become progressively more aware of your body's parts and allow them to express themselves freely in whatever ways seem natural. (For example, your left shoulder sags, or there is discomfort in the lower back.) Patients who are also being treated by osteopathic physicians report that these procedures may bring up vivid memories from their lives that are embedded in particular muscles or organs and conveyed through the central nervous system. If the memories are painful, they may generate strong emotions that are occasionally manifested in weeping, nausea, or depression. As a result, doctors use this procedure for limited periods (especially with young patients) with consultation from osteopathic physicians and other professionals who supervise it carefully. It is, however, a technique of great use in enhancing the patient's sense of body awareness.

Taking In More Space

Vision therapy aims at training you to "see more space," to take in a larger amount of space and more objects within it, through special exercises and the use of therapeutic lenses. Vision therapy doctors prescribe "stress-reducing" low-plus lenses for their patients as a tool for learning to take in more space. A plus lens is convex and gently pushes the point of focus farther away, enabling your eyes to see things in a wider perspective and giving them a cushion of distance that almost always relieves the stress of close work. Vision therapy has demonstrated that the greater volume of space you can take in through your eyes, the more information you will have for judging the spatial relationships of objects within your field of vision, and therefore the more accurately and efficiently you will be able to assimilate their meaning and act wisely in your own interests.

When you first increase your intake of space, you may see less clearly than before. But when you "hold on" to the new volume and work hard at improving your perception of the forms and structure within your enlarged "space world," you will achieve greater breadth of vision and greater acuity. The ultimate objective is to be able to concentrate on one central task, yet be simultaneously aware of all the ramifications and implications surrounding that central point. In the physical sense, this means broadening your field of vision. In the intellectual sense, it means understanding a wider network of relationships.

Behavioral optometrists do not necessarily view nearsightedness (myopia), or a particular bodily posture, as absolutely unchangeable. The two are mirror images of each other, reflections of an interlocking balance to which your body has gravitated in response to the multiple pressures imposed by your particular life. Both can be changed, but one cannot be changed without corresponding changes in the other.

Teaching you to take in a large volume of space is a central element of vision therapy. Activities to teach you to take in more space and thus enlarge your field of vision include Thumb Pursuits, the Wolff Wand, Pencil and Straw, and Two Sticks. These are described in Chapter 10.

Perception of Constant Size

Another reason why vision therapy emphasizes taking in more space relates to something called size constancy. People with efficient vision see objects in constant size at varying distances, mostly because vision is a function of the brain.

The point here is that we do not judge the size of an object just by the size of its image on our retina. If we did, everything close would appear too big,

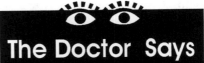

The Doctor Says

Some scientists have recently suggested that ADHD appears to be related to a magnocellular or M-Cell deficit in the visual centers of the brain. M-Cells are involved with our peripheral vision.

—Stan Appelbaum, OD, FCOVD

and everything far away would appear too small compared with the reality. This means that, through our visual system (the interaction of our eyes and brain), we alter our retinal image in accordance with our stored sensory experiences, to create a mental image of what is out there. We then mentally project that image out into space, and that is what we see. If our visual system is efficient, the size of the image we project will be consistent with the true size of the object—almost regardless of how close or far away the real object is. This is another classic example of the inextricable linkage between the eyes, the brain, the mind, and the experience stored in the body/mind system that is retrievable as memory.

Taking in "more space" is important to the achievement of size constancy, because when you take in more space you enhance your peripheral vision, and it is peripheral vision that provides the frame for what you see with your central vision. The strength and efficiency of your peripheral vision permit you to judge the true size of, and thus the true spatial relationships between, the various objects in the central field. You cannot have good peripheral vision if your eyes are narrowly channeled and focused close in, nor can you achieve size constancy under such conditions.

This is easily demonstrated by this simple procedure. Roll a sheet of paper into a tube and look through it with one eye. You will discover that, as you reduce the diameter of the tube, objects far away get much smaller, while near objects assume grotesquely large dimensions. This happens because, as you reduce the diameter of the tube, you reduce the available field of vision and thus your ability to organize what you "see" through your total visual-brain system. You become increasingly dependent on the image size reflected on the retina.

An exercise specifically designed to test and strengthen your perception of size constancy is known as the String Procedure and is described in Chapter 10.

Lens Therapy

We have mentioned lenses quite a bit throughout this book. Now we will talk about them in more detail.

Lenses are the most potent vision therapy tool, and should be used for every vision therapy patient. They are used both to improve eyesight and to improve vision. Remember, developmental/behavioral optometrists differentiate between our "eyesight" and our "vision." Eyesight is seeing the small letters on the doctor's letter chart, street signs, or what the teacher is writing on the whiteboard or blackboard. Vision is our ability to attend to, focus on, and comprehend what we see. Vision begins with eyesight, but it is much more than eyesight. You can have 20/20 eyesight and still have a vision problem. Good visual skills are something we can learn, and vision problems are at least potentially repairable.

Lenses can be either positive (plus) or negative (minus), which either magnify or minimize what we see. The same lens can be used for traditional, corrective, *compensatory* purposes for one person and for *therapeutic* purposes for someone else undergoing vision therapy. It all depends on the diagnosis and treatment plan.

If you are nearsighted (myopic), most optometrists will prescribe minus lenses, which bring your point of focus closer by compressing the volume of space your eyes can take in. This will improve your sharpness and clarity, but it will also narrow your scope of vision—your peripheral or side vision—and has the effect of "bringing the whole world into your lap," as Dr. Appelbaum has expressed it.

Depending on their strength or power, minus lenses provide the kind of vision you use when you aim a rifle: it is clear and sharp, but narrowly concentrated, and it produces stress for just those reasons. By reducing your field of vision, minus lenses also reduce your capacity to absorb an experience visually. By overemphasizing central vision and neglecting peripheral vision, they can adversely affect your bodily balance and general coordination. It is your peripheral vision that provides the frame or context for the objects you see;

without it, you experience difficulty in locating yourself precisely in space. Therefore, any attempt to "correct" myopic vision with procedures that further restrict your field of vision will in turn narrow your overall perception, with negative implications for brain activity and personality. This is the reason why all lenses must be prescribed very carefully. A careful balance must be achieved between the lens, which allows easy viewing of the blackboard or whiteboard or driving at night, and the entire eye/mind/brain connection.

If immediately clearer eyesight is the sole or primary goal, and minus lenses are prescribed, you will reduce the amount of space you take in and will therefore remain embedded or ingrained in your old visual habits, becoming progressively more and more nearsighted.

In vision therapy, the approach is very different. It aims at reducing myopia, not by bringing about immediate 20/20 acuity, but by training you to "see more space," to take in a larger volume of space and more objects within it, and to enhance the ability of your eyes and brain to focus objects both near and far. Having parents or grandparents who are very nearsighted or myopic means there is always a hereditary predisposition for the children to need glasses. The degree of myopia and whether the glasses continue to get stronger and stronger every year, is as much, if not more, a result of the environment and the development of good visual skills and abilities as it is hereditary.

Behavioral optometrists prescribe plus lenses for their patients as a tool for learning—to take in more space. A plus lens is convex and gently pushes the point of focus farther away, enabling your eyes to see things in a wider perspective and giving them a cushion of distance that almost always relieves the stress of close work. Vision therapy has demonstrated that the greater volume of space you can take in through your eyes, the more information you will have for judging the spatial relationships of objects within your field of vision, and therefore the more accurately and efficiently you will be able to assimilate their meaning and act accordingly.

Traditional, compensatory lenses are used by all eye doctors to sharpen what we see by reducing blur. Therapeutic lenses, on the other hand, help our *visual process* improve itself. Therapeutic lenses require us to use our visual system more intensively and to adjust it more finely. Optometrists who are board certified in vision therapy (fellows) of the College of Optometrists in Vision Development (www.covd.org), are much more likely than traditional eye doctors to use therapeutic lenses.

Lenses are usually the decisive factor in a successful vision therapy program. They must be carefully prescribed and adjusted at various stages of the program to ensure they are moving the patient in the desired direction, without undue stress.

Your visual system is the master coordinator of your mind/body system. Changing your vision with lenses forces you to adjust your posture, your coordination, and all bodily and mental functions affected by your central and autonomic nervous systems. The power and importance of lenses are the principal reasons why vision therapy cannot be a do-it-yourself program, but requires the initial diagnosis and continuing guidance of a developmental optometrist who is board certified in vision therapy. For more information, go to: www.visionhelp.com, www.covd.org, and www.aoa.org.

How Do Lenses Work?

Basically, lenses alter the way you see the world. *Traditional, compensatory lenses* do not correct or cure reduced eyesight, they merely make up for it. They compensate for a refractive error in your visual system, whether the trouble is nearsightedness (myopia), farsightedness (hyperopia), irregular shape of the cornea or other surfaces of the eye (astigmatism), two eyes that focus at significantly different distances (anisometropia), or cross-eye (strabismus). Compensatory lenses are put in conventional spectacles or contacts and are usually worn all the time. The assumption is that you cannot see satisfactorily without them, and that nothing else can be done to correct your underlying visual deficiency.

Behavioral optometrists, on the other hand, believe that functional visual deficiencies can be wholly or partially corrected with the help of therapeutic lenses. ***Therapeutic lenses*** help bring about corrective changes and improvements in your eyes, and help your whole body/mind system work toward better alignment and coordination. Behavioral optometrists use therapeutic lenses in two ways: for rehabilitation or for development. For *rehabilitation*, therapeutic lenses are most often used when your eyes are poorly coordinated (they may focus at different distances) and when this inefficiency causes stress or bodily clumsiness.

Therapeutic lenses are usually low powered, worn for special activities like reading or sports, and for relatively short periods of time. The lens prescriptions are changed after your visual system has made an adjustment in the desired direction, and they are changed frequently as a means of pushing you further along the path to correction and better alignment. When the overall correction has been achieved, there is frequently no more need for therapeutic lenses.

Developmental lenses are used almost exclusively with children, for two purposes: (1) to guide and reinforce visual development in a child who has—through some accident or trauma—missed a step in the pattern of normal visual development, and (2) to control the development of vision during the school years in an effort to prevent abnormal conditions like myopia or strabismus. Used for these purposes, the lenses are sometimes called preventive lenses. The rationale for developmental lenses can be explained by comparing our eyes with our hands and feet. We wear shoes to protect our feet from cold and hard pavements. When we play baseball, we wear a protective glove that makes it easier to catch the ball. Why then should we not try to protect our children's visual systems, which are at least as precious and important?

How Close Work Can Cause Myopia

Now we will demonstrate how we use the plus lens to help with the widespread condition of myopia (nearsightedness). First, let us do some explaining. Myopia is a widespread phenomenon in our society, which is still paper-oriented but also computer-driven, and very rapidly becoming electronically based. Our peripheral and distance vision are being sacrificed as we read and work day in and day out with the help of computers—whose display screens have gotten smaller and smaller—and hand-held devices such as cell phones, iPods, and Blackberries.

Sustained close work of any kind can lead to myopia, because it requires a narrow intensity of focus. There are several fascinating truths about the physical aspects of reading and thinking that reinforce our belief that the images we see in our field of vision are the building blocks of our reasoning power.

Vision is a symbolizing process, which means we label an object with a word. Speech and thought are symbolizing processes too. Therefore, when you read the word *cow*, your mind leaps away from the page to your image of the animal. When you do this, tests show that you actually focus through and beyond the page to visualize the cow. Your memory has been triggered by the word—the symbol.

But success in schoolwork, or in any other intellectual task, requires us to simultaneously see the language symbols and translate them into meaningful terms. We need flexible eyes for this and the visual skills and abilities to enable us to literally see in two places at one time. Tests show that this requires a highly developed ability to control the focus of our eyes, to shift quickly and easily back and forth between the short focus on the word itself, and the longer focus on the idea and meaning beyond the word.

This ability relates directly to the fact that intense close work is linked to nearsightedness (myopia). Beginning readers focus on the words and phrases. They take in these language symbols but do not visualize their meaning. In order to comprehend the symbols, readers must push the focus of the eye through the word, and through and beyond the page. When this process is pursued intensively and over a long period of time, it can lead to myopia. This is because your struggle to comprehend—to translate word symbols into genuine meaning—causes your visual system to close in, to focus more sharply on the central object, as if you were aiming a rifle. When this occurs, your system tends to go rigid. Your eye focus gets narrow and fixed, and your neck and back stiffen.

Both your peripheral and distance vision are neglected in your effort to focus all available energy on the complicated problem of mastering the intellectual symbols in front of you.

The Plus Lens

In 1959, Dr. Darrell Boyd Harmon demonstrated that using a simple low plus lens can reduce the physiological stress in our mind/body system when we are engaged in problem solving involving our eyes and brain. This gave scientific verification to what had been observed in clinical practice for many years. Since then, the low plus lens has become a special tool of vision therapy, used not only to give immediate relief from visual stress but also to provide protection against beginning myopia for persons whose jobs involve a large amount of close work, reading, computer use, or analytical reading.

A plus lens is convex; therefore, it spreads the image across a wider area of your retina. This helps you take in more space and enhances your peripheral vision. As vision therapy patients improve their vision, many will benefit from plus lenses. When their visual coordination improves, the doctor prescribes low plus lenses for near work, to improve their vision, not their eyesight. This helps them sustain their newly acquired near point efficiency without constricting into myopia. Patients being brought out of myopia through vision therapy need a plus lens to support their new ability to converge their eyes at a greater distance. Plus lenses frequently permit them to continue their newly efficient visual processing without going into the constriction of myopia.

The need for low plus lens reading glasses is therefore a sign of progress and improvement. The specific power of the lens is determined by the doctor's measurement of how the visual system aligns and how the visual sustaining skills are affected.

Some Case Histories

The following case histories illustrate the important role of low plus lenses.

Michelle

Michelle had eye muscle (strabismus) surgery when she was 8 years old. The operation was for the resection of the left inferior oblique muscle (the muscle responsible for elevating the eye and turning it in). As a result of the surgery, Michelle tilted her head at an extreme angle, virtually laying it against her left shoulder. This condition persisted for 4 years until her parents, in despair, brought her to a vision therapy optometrist when she was 12 years old.

The optometrist found that the basic problem was a severe "alternating hypertropia," which is an uncontrollable tendency of first one eye, and then the other, to gaze upward at a sharp angle. The right eye was worse than the left, but both eyes tended to jump up and down in the course of reading. Michelle instinctively tilted her head to eliminate the effort required to lower the right eye. With the head tilted, she did not have to pull it down, but could gaze more or less horizontally at the target. She was also nearsighted (myopic). She held her head in her left hand while reading. She read slowly and with low comprehension and short attention span. Although she was already in a special class for slow learners, she remained nervous, irritable, inattentive, and obviously stressed whenever she had to read for more than a few minutes. She read primarily with her right eye. Michelle was diagnosed with attention deficit hyperactivity disorder (ADHD) and was given stimulant medication to improve her attention.

The doctor used therapeutic lenses to teach Michelle, with each of her eyes separately, to focus on an object at various distances, since the basic problem was that each eye tended to see a given object at a different distance. To avoid the confusion caused by this inaccurate processing of information, Michelle unconsciously blocked out one eye most of the time. She was referred to an occupational therapist to begin a sensory integration treatment program.

During the first 3 months of vision therapy, there was no change in Michelle's condition. Then one day, she saw both eyes in a mirror at a distance of 6 feet, using a therapeutic device called "Polaroid lenses." This indicated she was now using both eyes, rather than suppressing one eye or the other. After 4 months of vision therapy, she began to hold her head erect while reading. After 5 months, she had virtually eliminated the tilt and was doing homework without apparent strain. The hypertropia at far distance was gone. The eyes still tended to move upward, but Michelle could now control this by mental effort and mild muscular exertion, and she was able to reduce her medication used to improve her attention. For the first time, Michelle started reading for pleasure without eyestrain. After 6 months, the doctor prescribed bifocals (a plus .75 lens for near work to improve her vision and regular, compensatory glasses for distance to improve her eyesight) to ease the nearsightedness. The occupational therapy together with the vision therapy was allowing both sides of Michelle's body and both of her eyes to work together as a team.

By the 7th month of therapy, Michelle's reading and writing had greatly improved. During the 9th month, she began to ride a two-wheel bicycle for the first time, which had been nearly impossible when her head was tilted. This meant she had now achieved a much better balance of her whole mind/ body system. After the 12th month, she was a well-organized child, showing good physical coordination and able to play fast-moving games. She was less and less dependent on her lenses. The doctor felt Michelle was approaching the "stabilization phase," which signals the logical completion of vision therapy. The combination of optometric vision therapy and sensory integration occupational therapy made a significant difference in Michelle's ability to not only do well in school, but also in her self-confidence on the playground and the ball field.

Amanda

Amanda was a college student who had worn contact lenses through high school without any change in prescription. But in college she began to suffer from severe headaches and tension around her eyes. She also felt she was "overfocusing," meaning that she saw too much detail close in, but nothing much beyond 5 feet. She sensed this was producing not only a visual but also a psychological and intellectual restriction.

She went to a developmental optometrist who gave her a set of plus glasses to wear over the contact lenses, which reduced the net lens power. This immediately reduced the tension, enlarged her field of vision, and soon caused a shift to a more comfortable visual postural balance. Over the next 11 months, the doctor made progressive changes in both the contact lenses and the glasses, gradually reducing the net lens power by nearly 80 percent, as shown in the chart.

Appointment	Contact Lens	Glasses	Net Lens Power
1	-3.75		-3.75
2	-3.25	+0.50	-2.75
3	-2.75	+0.75	-2.00
4	-2.75	+1.25	-1.50
5	-2.50	+1.50	-1.00

As a result of wearing therapeutic lenses that forced her to take in a greater volume of space, Amanda lost her tension and her headaches. She achieved a broader visual and also a broader psychological comprehension, and found her college studies easier to grasp and complete. "I write with greater facility now, and can actually see how sentences should be constructed."

Procedures You Can Try at Home

Now we want to show you some of the procedures to be done at home that are part of a vision therapy program. They are simple and interesting, and involve little or no equipment and no lenses. Try them at home, and if you notice vision improvement by doing these simple activities, imagine all the benefits you might get by working with a doctor!

Optometrists do not always agree on how to implement specific vision therapy techniques, but they all agree on the fundamental purpose. Procedures designed to improve your vision can temporarily change your vision, but to get permanent vision improvement, you must achieve true vision changes— meaning changes in how your brain processes and interprets visual information. This is done by developing and improving your fundamental visual skills and abilities.

Remember, that not much happens if you do vision therapy without a doctor's guidance. Vision therapy is not just eye exercise. Unlike other forms of exercise, the goal of vision therapy is not to strengthen eye muscles. The eye muscles in the vast majority of vision therapy patients are already strong enough to do anything they have to do.

Throughout this book we have emphasized that full benefits can be realized only within the context of a treatment program personally prescribed by a professional optometrist, who is board certified in vision therapy, who has examined your eyes and diagnosed your problem, and who provides direct supervision, assessment, and guidance.

The training is a process involving self-monitoring and self-correcting by you, the patient. The doctor and therapist will help you learn to monitor your own visual process. In this way, you will discover the consistencies and mismatches in your personal style of processing visual information, but what you

The Doctor Says

The patient does the self-correcting self-monitoring. The doctor is the "coach."

—Stan Appelbaum, OD, FCOVD

do with this new knowledge will be mostly up to you. Your motivation to change is crucial.

Now, on to the procedures!

Body Awareness Procedures

The following activities are designed to improve body awareness, balance, and coordination. They are called the Ballet, the Balance Rail, and Bilateral Motor Equivalents.

Ballet

A simple activity to increase body awareness, balance, flexibility, and control is called the Ballet. It is done by covering one eye with an eye patch. (Before using an eye patch, check with your eye doctor to make sure it is okay.) In bare or sock feet, you stand in a comfortable posture, directing your line of sight to a point 20 or 30 feet in front of you. Holding that target, you slowly raise your left leg in front of you, as high and as straight as possible. Then you slowly lower it, but without letting the foot touch the ground. Then raise it in the same way to the side and lower it again without allowing the foot to touch the ground. Then you raise the leg behind you and slowly return it to the ground. Next, repeat the exercise with the right leg. You then shift the eye patch to the other eye and perform the procedure with first the left and then the right leg (see illustration). Finally, you perform the exercise with both eyes covered or closed.

Initially, most people discover they have far less control over their bodies than they thought, and have particular trouble visualizing the room and the position

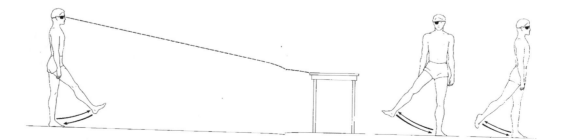

of their bodies in it when both eyes are covered. It is especially difficult to visualize the area behind you.

Like the standing awareness we described in the Chapter 8, the Ballet is designed to develop and enhance your sense of body awareness and control, and your sense of spatial orientation, by increasing awareness and helping you to concentrate on the two primary centers of gravity—your pelvic area and the middle of the chest. Binocular mismatches cannot be corrected by simply concentrating harder with the eyes. First, you need better balance and alignment throughout the body/mind system. Body awareness is key to improved posture, and both are essential to improve the efficiency with which your visual system processes information—that is, achieves a more accurate matching of visual perception with the true characteristics of objects in the physical world. To improve our visual performance, we must alter the way we use our bodies by moving toward a balanced, ideal position. This balanced posture implies balancing our bodies in all dimensions.

Balance Rail

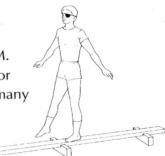

Behavioral optometrists tell the story of their mentor, Dr. A.M. Skeffington, the pioneer in this specialty, who was waiting for his train at the railroad station of a small Midwestern town many years ago. For diversion, he started walking on one of the railroad tracks to see if he could balance himself. After a while he came upon a young girl doing the same thing, approaching him on the same rail. They looked each other straight in the eye and continued forward. Just before they met, both stepped off the track to allow the other to pass. As the girl stepped off, Dr. Skeffington noted that she went "from straight-eyed to strabismic"—that is, to cross-eyed. From this, he deduced that she was normally cross-eyed, but when she was forced to maintain bodily balance on the rail, her eyes had temporarily straightened out. This observation strengthened Dr. Skeffington's view that vision is malleable, and that good visual performance depends on a harmonious alignment between eyes and body. His judgment led to the widespread use of a 4-inch Balance Rail or

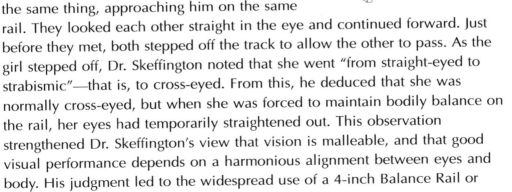

walking rail (mounted a few inches off the ground) as a basic device in vision therapy.

You walk on the Balance Rail in sock feet with one eye patched and the other eye trying to take in as much space and as many objects as possible. You quickly discover that keeping in view multiple reference points, simultaneously, gives you a much more stable balance than if you fix your eye on only one point. You locate your body more accurately and precisely by reference to several objects in your field of vision than by reference to only one of them. You walk both forward and backward on the Balance Rail. And when you have mastered it with first one and then the other eye covered, you try to master it with both eyes covered. The key to success in this last variation is to visualize the reference points in the room as you remember them, and to concentrate mainly on "centering" your balance in your abdomen and lower chest.

The Balance Rail is used in many regular and special educational schools. Sometimes a tilted board is used.

Bilateral Motor Equivalents

The set of exercises known as Bilateral Motor Equivalents is designed to reduce the pronounced tendency in each of us to left or right "sidedness." Our

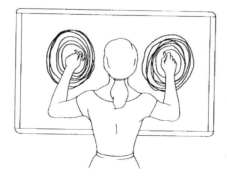

bodies are an interacting complex of subsystems mediated by vision and the brain. Each bodily movement is normally directed by or through the dominant "side," but each movement always involves a counterbalancing movement by the other, nonpreferred side. The counterbalancing movement is often weak or awkward because we have done nothing to develop strength or agility on the nonpreferred side.

A series of activities were devised in which you draw large circles on a chalkboard, first with the dominant hand, then with the nonpreferred hand, and then with both hands simultaneously in a variety of clockwise and counterclockwise movements. Using the same principle, you can carry out a number of ordinary tasks—for example, buttoning your shirt, shaving, eating, and dialing a telephone—using the "wrong" or nonpreferred hand. Diligent practice will bring you a far more even-handed dexterity and in turn better balance and coordinate your whole body/mind system.

Making counterclockwise circles on a whiteboard or chalkboard is also helpful to improve handwriting. Our language involves making counterclockwise circles when we write, and combining this procedure with occupational therapy techniques like "Handwriting Without Tears" can be very beneficial for children with handwriting issues.

Taking In More Space

The following procedures, designed to help you develop and to take in more space and therefore enlarge your field of vision, are called Thumb Pursuits, the Wolff Wand, Two Sticks, and Pencil and Straw.

Thumb Pursuits

Thumb Pursuits is a widely used vision therapy procedure that is deceptively simple. Start by standing erect, covering your right eye with an eye patch or with your left hand, and then following the upright thumb of your right hand with your right eye as you move your thumb slowly in a random pattern, in and out, up, down, and around. Do the same exercise with the other eye.

The basic aim of this exercise is to see the thumb while simultaneously extending your eye's coverage to as many other objects and as much space in the room as possible. Try to achieve a clear focus on the thumb in the near distance and at the same time a clear focus on other objects farther away.

As you perform these home procedures, ask yourself the following questions:

- Can I see the thumb clearly at all positions within the reach of my arm? If not, at what positions and distance is it blurred?

- When my thumb is clear and sharp, is the rest of the room also in focus, or is it blurred?
- If I move my posture toward the ideal upright balanced position, does this help to keep both my thumb and the rest of the room in simultaneous focus?
- Conversely, if I deliberately slump, how does that affect my ability to focus?
- How much space can I take in at one time? If I try to maximize the amount, how does this affect the clarity with which I see my thumb or other specific objects?
- How can I improve clarity in the central area without losing the amount of space I see?
- How can I improve clarity in my left and right peripheries without losing the amount of space I see?
- Does my thumb vary in size as I move it in and out, or does it remain constant? Do I see any advantage in having it remain a constant size?

How you answer these questions begins to define your present visual performance, meaning the amount of space you can take in and the amount of control you have under varying distances, focus points, and postures. At the beginning, most patients have trouble achieving a simultaneous clarity of their thumb and the background objects. Most will lose clarity of the thumb if they stretch their eyes to take in a greater amount of space. Most will have only limited peripheral vision. Most will see their thumb grow bigger or smaller as it moves closer or farther away from their eyes.

The Thumb Pursuit is therefore a useful introduction to the truth that the moving thumb exists not in isolation, but within a three-dimensional world comprising you, your total field of vision, and all other objects within that field. How well you organize that total volume of space will determine how clearly you see the thumb. The more reference points you see clearly, the more accurately you will fix the thumb target in space. Children and adults with attention deficit hyperactivity disorder (ADHD), other attention problems, and learning difficulties related to their vision, often have problems doing this simple procedure.

Wolff Wand

A variation of the Thumb Pursuit is the Wolff Wand (named for its inventor, Dr. Bruce Wolff of Cincinnati, Ohio), in which a small steel ball bearing mounted on a metal wand is manipulated, by either the patient or the doctor. A silver teaspoon or tablespoon serves equally well. This exercise is particularly well adapted to stretching and therefore enhancing your peripheral vision, since the wand can be moved to either side as far as your arm extends (and should normally be moved in an irregular pattern, both back and forth and at varying distances from your eyes; see illustration). It is important to see peripheral objects clearly, rather than merely being aware of their existence, because they provide the frame of the picture and therefore give clarity to the objects in your central field of vision. The clarity of the central target is proportionate to the clarity of the peripheral field.

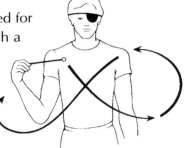

The basic objective of both the Thumb Pursuit and the Wolff Wand tracking procedure is to teach you to follow a target smoothly and easily with the eyes, and to know where the target is in space. Because the target is continually changing its location (often on all three planes simultaneously), you are constantly required to make different spatial calculations in a three-dimensional world. This involves you in what behavioral optometrists call "accommodative rock," which has nothing to do with music. It refers to your eye's ability to shift smoothly from near to far focus and vice versa. These activities, like a number of others, also teach you that your own body is the center and basic frame of reference for all of your judgments about objects in your field of vision.

What you see depends not only on where but also on how you stand. The ability to process visual information centrally or peripherally, and the ease of shifting this ability as the task demands, is a fundamental goal of any successful vision therapy treatment program.

As we said in Chapter 8, learning to take in a greater amount of visual space is an important part of vision therapy. The more space you can take in, the more accurately you can see the objects in spatial relationship to one another. And the more clearly you can distinguish those objects (their different shapes and textures), the better you can interpret and utilize the vital information they provide.

The higher the level of your visual performance, the greater physical and mental efficiency you will achieve—you will read better, enjoy reading more, think faster, and much, much more.

In reading, the practical advantages of being able to take in a larger volume of space and to be aware of the precise location of objects within it are obvious. Reading depends on the information you grasp in a given moment. How much volume you see in that time determines what you can supply to your brain in order to get meaning from a printed page. Accordingly, if your perceived volume within that moment includes a whole phrase, a whole sentence, or several sentences, you will be a more efficient reader than the person who can absorb, during the same moment, only a word or two.

The same argument applies even more to driving a car, which is a survival process. Our lives literally depend sometimes on how much information we can absorb in a split second.

The Doctor Says

Vision therapy is fitness training for your eye muscles. It is a re-education program for your eyes, mind, and brain. And, just like learning to ride a bike, once you teach your eye muscles how to work their best, they don't forget.

—Bryce Appelbaum, OD

But volume alone is obviously not the only advantage. It does you no good to see a large area of the printed page if you cannot see clearly enough to identify the words quickly and without strain. Similarly, an ability to see the horizon beyond the highway will not help if you cannot identify the moving vehicles in your immediate vicinity and what they are doing. To be useful, the ability to take in a larger volume must be accompanied by a high level of accuracy.

Greater volume combined with clarity is therefore a basic aim of the training, and procedures like Thumb Pursuits and the Wolff Wand can assist in its realization.

Two Sticks

This excellent procedure involves two round sticks or dowels, each about 24 inches long, one held in each hand. With one eye covered, you bring the sticks together from various distances and various angles (see illustration). The purpose is to test how much space you can "control" in terms of accurate depth perception horizontally, vertically, and diagonally. Standing straight, you hold the sticks so that one is extended farther than the other and their tips are several inches apart.

You next determine the specific point in space where you believe the tips of the sticks will touch if you moved them toward each other. You then move both sticks quickly to that point. In the beginning you will miss frequently, even from a distance of only a few inches. One stick will be higher or lower, and the two ends will pass in space instead of touching. If you miss, it means you have not sufficiently organized your field of vision—by fixing the central objects in relation to objects in the background and on the peripheries, or it means your hand-eye coordination is faulty. It may reflect deficiencies in both of these areas. You should note that not only space but also space/time is involved in this exercise.

You should immediately correct the error by bringing the stick ends together, and then repeat the exercise from the same distance several times—as many times as are required to perfect your depth perception and your eye-hand coordination at that distance.

Next, do the same thing with the other eye patched or covered. Then widen the starting distance between the sticks and vary the angle of approach. And do it again. It is a procedure of wide variations and great training value especially if you are recovering from an acquired brain injury. People who have had a stroke or traumatic brain injury should seek the guidance of an optometrist who specializes in this area. For more information, contact the Neuro-Optometric Rehabilitation Association (www.NORA.cc).

Pencil and Straw

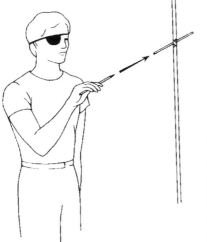

A variation of the Two Sticks activity involves a pencil and a hollow drinking straw. Tape the straw horizontally at the center, to any freestanding vertical that will permit a clear approach from either side, such as an open doorway. Then, with one eye covered, hold the pencil in your left hand 12 to 18 inches from the left end of the straw (or in your right hand the same distance from the right end). The object is to line up the pencil and the straw, perceiving them as a single horizontal line and judging for depth perception. You then move the pencil in a single swift motion in an effort to run the pencil tip inside the straw (see illustration).

As in the Two Sticks activity, you will probably miss frequently in the beginning, moving the pencil slightly above or below the straw, or slightly behind or in front of it. Correct each error immediately, and repeat until you have achieved perfect eye-hand control of this space/time relationship.

Size Constancy

The following activity, designed to test and enhance your perception of size constancy, is known as the String Procedure.

String Procedure

Sensing the size of a particular object accurately at varying distances in space is not easy or automatic. But as we explained in Chapter 8, your perception of constant size is an important measure of your visual efficiency. It depends, first of all, on your knowing how much space the object occupies. It also depends on your ability to organize your field of vision—to see all the objects within it, including those on both peripheries, and to judge accurately the distances between each of them and the central target object, as well as the distance of each of the objects from you.

The String Procedure illustrates this problem and challenge. With one eye covered, you stand in the center of the room holding a piece of string 4 or 5 feet long stretched out between your hands. You look around and pick any amount of distance you think is within the span of your outstretched arms—for example, the width of a bureau. You then ask yourself how far apart you have to hold your hands to make the distance between them agree exactly with the width of the bureau. You then adjust your hands on the string and move to the bureau to see if your estimate is correct (see illustration). Most people fail this test at first. If you pass it, you already have a reasonably good sense of size constancy.

But the harder part of the exercise comes next. You correct the length of string to match the width of the bureau. You then back away slowly, trying simultaneously to maintain a visual match between the bureau and the string. You try to see how far you can back away before the string no longer appears to match the width of the bureau. At that point, you should stop, take a deep breath, and begin to apply the fundamentals of vision therapy.

In essence, your challenge is to organize your field of vision: (a) assume an erect posture, as close as possible to the ideal; (b) take in as much volume of space as possible in the room, being sharply aware of objects on the periphery and judging their distance from each other and from the bureau; and (c) determine how much volume each of the peripheral objects occupies (this involves a judgment as to the true size of each). This procedure takes practice and more practice, as well as considerable tears and sweat. It cannot be mastered immediately. Gradually, however, you will discover that, as you become more aware of the precise information contained in your field of vision, your sense of size constancy will improve.

More Home Procedures

Here are several excellent procedures you may encounter in some vision therapy doctor's offices. These activities will help not only your vision but also your balance, coordination, and performance. A procedure using a rubber ball suspended from the ceiling by a string to help improve your visual skills in several areas is called the Marsden Ball Technique.

Marsden Ball Technique

This exercise (invented by Dr. Carl Marsden of Rocky Ford, Colorado) starts by suspending a rubber ball from the ceiling down to the level of your chest or chin. In the original exercise, the ball was swung in a circle or an arc, and the patient followed it with both eyes open or with one eye covered. It was a simple pursuit procedure designed to require the muscles of the eye to relax and contract as the distance between the eye and the ball was lengthened and shortened. Like the Wolff Wand and Thumb Pursuits, the purpose of this exercise was to develop "accommodative rock," meaning the ability of the eye to shift smoothly from near to far focus and vice versa.

The Marsden Ball Technique has been developed and refined over the years, and now frequently encompasses a whole series of procedures that range from simple to quite difficult and sophisticated.

In one variation, letters of the alphabet are attached to the ball, and you are instructed to call out the letters you see as the ball moves through its circle or arc. In another variation, you hold a pencil beside your ear, like a dart. You then attempt, in a swift thrust, to hit the moving ball at various positions on the arc.

To test eye-hand coordination and to engage the whole body in rhythmic movement in relation to the moving ball, some practitioners have enhanced the exercise by adding a basket, 3 or 4 inches deep and about the size of a small salad bowl. You hold the basket in both hands and move it beneath the moving ball, trying to keep the ball inside of, but not touching, the basket. As the ball swings in its circle, your whole body moves rhythmically with it, except for your feet, which remain comfortably planted. You look like someone doing a stationary waltz—you are in fact exercising and refining the motor control that is the basis of superior eye-body coordination.

Eye Aerobics

Here are seven "eye aerobics" that Dr. Appelbaum uses with his patients:

1. Move your eyes upwards as far as you can, and then downwards as far as you can. Repeat four more times. Blink quickly a few times to relax your eye muscles.

2. Now do the same thing, using points to your right and to your left, at eye level. Keep your raised fingers or two pencils on each side as guides and adjust them so that you can see them clearly when moving the eyes to the right and to the left, but without straining. Keeping the fingers at eye level, and moving only the eyes, look to the right at your chosen point, then to the left. Repeat four times. Blink several times, then close your eyes and rest.

3. Choose a point you can see from the right corner of your eyes when you raise them, and another that you can see from the left corner of your eyes when you lower them, half closing the lids. Remember to retain your original posture: spine erect, hands on knees, head straight and motionless. Look at your chosen point in the right corner up, then to the one in the left corner down. Repeat four times. Blink several times. Close your eyes and rest. Now do the same exercise in reverse. That is, first look to the left corner up, then to the right corner down. Repeat four times. Blink several times. Close the eyes and rest.

4. This eye aerobic should ideally be done 3 or 4 days after you have begun the above procedures. Slowly roll your eyes first clockwise, then counterclockwise as follows. Lower your eyes and look at the floor, then slowly move the eyes to the left, higher and higher until you see the ceiling. Now continue circling to the right, lower and lower down, until you see the floor again. Do this slowly, making a full-vision circle. Blink, close your eyes, and rest. Then repeat the same action counterclockwise. Do this five times, then blink the eyes for at least 5 seconds. When rolling the eyes, make as large a circle as possible, so that you feel a little strain as you do the exercise. This stretches the eye muscles to the maximum extent, giving better results.

5. Next comes a changing-vision procedure. While doing it you alternately shift your vision from close to distant points several times. Take a pencil, or use your finger, and hold it under the tip of your nose. Then start moving it away, without raising it, until you have fixed it at the closest possible distance where you can see it clearly without any blur. Then raise your eyes a little, look straight into the distance and there find a small point that you can also see very clearly. Now look at the closer point—the pencil or your finger tip—then shift to the farther point in the distance. Repeat several times, blink, close your eyes, and squeeze them tight.

6. Close your eyes as tightly as you possibly can. Really squeeze the eyes, so the eye muscles contract. Hold this contraction for 3 seconds, and then let go quickly. This procedure causes a deep relaxation of the eye muscles, and is especially beneficial after the slight strain caused by doing the above procedures. Blink your eyes a few times.

7. This procedure is called "palming" and is very relaxing to the eyes. It was first described by William Bates, M.D., in his 1940 book and is helpful in preserving your visual skills and abilities. Palming also seems to have a beneficial, relaxing effect on the nervous system. It is an ideal way to finish off these eye aerobics. This exercise is good for immediate relief of eyestrain, fatigue, and headaches related to excessive visual concentration. Mary Kawar, a highly regarded occupational therapist

practicing in El Cerrito (Berkeley), California, teaches this exercise to doctors and therapists across the country.

Sit in a chair with both elbows on a table in a comfortable position. Keeping your eyes open, cup your hands over your eyes so no light can be seen. It is important that there are no light leaks, so you might have to squeeze your fingers together. Hold this comfortable position for at least 5 to 10 minutes while breathing deeply. Your eyes and whole body will become rested in a very short time. The idea is to look into complete darkness while keeping your eyes open, breathing deeply.

8. "Thinker" activity—This excellent procedure was brought to our attention also by Mary Kawar. Sit with both elbows on the table and close your eyes. Hold your head with both hands in the position of the famous sculpture by Rodin, "The Thinker." While holding your head still, swing your eyes from side to side and from ear to ear with a firm, definitive motion for at least 5 minutes. This will help you recall details, names, important facts, and more!

9. Peripheral Vision Expansion activity—This variation of Dr. Larry McDonald's vision therapy chart (see below) is a good tool to increase your ability to take in a large volume of visual space to help you read more and faster with less effort and energy. Start by focusing on the dot at the center of the eye chart pictured below. Look only at the dot for 4 seconds. Use your side vision to begin looking at the four letters surrounding the dot. Begin focusing on the L and then the H and then the Y and then the E. Then focus on the next larger set of four letters in sequence: the T and then the A and S and P. Go to the next larger set of four letters: K, M, F, and N. Then Z, K, Y, and E. Again, V, T, Y, X. Next, L, N, T, and A. Finally, N, Y, U, and K.

Hold four letters of the same size all at once in your peripheral vision for 4 seconds, then the next largest letters for 4 seconds, and so on. The closer you hold the chart to your eyes, the harder it will be to expand your peripheral vision. The farther you hold the chart from your eyes, the easier it will be.

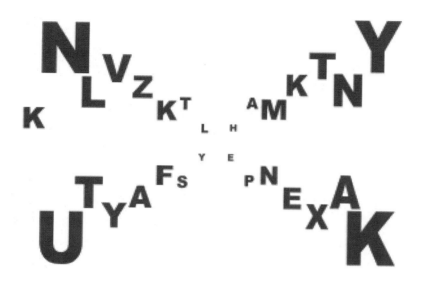

Infinity Walk

Children and adults who have learning, motor, or behavior problems that affect their vision benefit greatly from the Infinity Walk. The theory and method of this exercise were conceived in the mid-1980s by clinical psychotherapist Dr. Deborah Sunbeck. It is a highly effective way to get the whole body involved with the visual system.

The activity is both simple and profound. Basically, you walk in a figure eight pattern while looking at a specific object in the room—a visual target. This simple, repetitive movement is progressively refined, with tasks added to improve your skills.

Once they have practiced the Infinity Walk at home with a visual target, patients often become highly motivated to start the part of vision therapy that includes procedures that cannot be done at home and will take them even further in developing their visual and vestibular abilities.

The Infinity Walk often makes a huge difference very quickly with visual problems. Why should we expect our two eyes to work together if the rest of our body is not? Our two eyes are part of a whole body that has to be bilaterally integrated.

The Infinity Walk is a recognized clinical method not just in developmental optometry and vision therapy, but also occupational therapy, psychology, neurorehabilitation, and physical and sports medicine. Educators all over the world have brought the Infinity Walk to their schools and special education programs. When sensory, perceptual, language, cognitive, or relational tasks are added to the basic exercise, it can eventually produce positive change in the whole person, and many levels of growth. Infinity Walkers do not even need to walk to benefit from the method. For example, the Infinity Walk practice can be assisted by the use of a wheelchair, a baby stroller, or a parent's shoulder (in the case of an infant).

The Doctor Says

Glasses, contact lenses, medications, surgery, an eye patch— these are the only kinds of solutions that patients are expecting. So, I use procedures like Infinity Walk to prove a point. I teach them how to do Infinity Walk at home while looking at a visual target. When they come back to their next appointment, they're frequently not so tired after reading; the nausea in the car is reduced. Their symptoms are better. This tells them that they are part of the solution.

—Stan Appelbaum, OD, FCOVD

Nancy's Story

Nancy, a high school student, had many visual problems stemming from her early years in a Russian orphanage. Below she relates how she finally overcame her problems through vision therapy. In the process, she developed a passion for the ocular sciences and hopes to become an eye doctor.

Vision therapy has benefited me in two ways. It has improved my visual system tremendously, so much so that now I can now perform many near tasks. Second, it has cultivated my passion for the ocular sciences, ever since Dr. Appelbaum stimulated my curiosity during vision therapy sessions. Each session would revive my interest in the science behind what I was doing—the relationship between accommodation (focusing) and convergence (controlling my eyes).

In January 2003, I remember sitting at a restaurant in New York City and thinking to myself, I have to be an ophthalmologist, an optometrist, or both. Then I thought to myself, I have to get rid of this double vision.

I was adopted at age 3 from Russia. I was born premature, and my biological mother left me at the hospital. With few caretakers and many children, the orphanage did very little to stimulate my visual system. I never learned how to form a stereoscopic image, and no one knew I had more than three diopters of hyperopia (meaning that objects appeared blurry close, far, and everywhere in between).

The first thing my parents and sister did when they adopted me was to see if there was anything wrong with me physically. They came to the conclusion that my head was oversized, and that was it, until one Easter, I could not spot dyed eggs in green grass, and I had the habit of staring into space or at light fixtures when talking to other people.

My parents brought me to a pediatric ophthalmologist with 35 years' experience. He prescribed glasses for me and told my parents my eyes wandered outwards, but I tended to use my right eye much more than my left one. Over a period of 4 years or so, he gradually diminished my prescription and therefore forced my eyes to stay straight. This decrease in hyperopia is common: as the eye grows, many children end up not needing glasses. He gave me a cycloplegic exam every other visit, to make sure that my refractive error was really decreasing so rapidly. I remember that my ophthalmologist's news that I "didn't even need to wear glasses at all" coincided with a science project in school. Naturally, I decided to do a project on nearsightedness, farsightedness, and astigmatism.

A few years later, I went through a phase where I thought glasses were "cool." I told my parents I could not see just so I could go to the eye doctor and get the glasses I wanted. After many a time of hearing "Nancy's eyes are just fine," along with my nervous habit of giggling at the eye doctor's office, my parents, understandably, became blind (no pun intended) to my protests. During a 4th-grade required vision and hearing screening, the school told my parents that I ought to get my eyes evaluated. I was given a slightly different prescription and new frames.

Two years later, as the homework load became more demanding, I realized I was overcompensating for my vision. I became aware that I could read— mostly with my right eye—and I could see far away, but I could also "relax" my eyes and "let the image go blurry." I told my parents about this so that I would end up back in the doctor's chair. "Nancy, you know, the doctor can tell if you're faking. He has special techniques that measure the length of your eyeball. He knows when you're pretending to not be able to read the letters."

I giggled to myself. The ophthalmologist entered, and luckily he spared me the atropine drops. He asked me to read the letters on the Snellen Chart ("E" chart, which I had not quite memorized by then) and noticed my posture and eyestrain. "Relax your eyes." I relaxed them and looked at the white blur on the wall. I could not even make out the "E." (I had memorized that letter by then.) The ophthalmologist placed lenses in the measurable glasses and told me to read. After switching a few lenses, he realized that the closer the corrective lenses approached plano (no correction), the more I was accommodating and converging (straining my eyes). My eyesight was the same as when I came from the orphanage; my ciliary body (the muscles inside my eye) simply got strong enough to compensate for schoolwork with almost no correction. He sent us, with my original prescription, to the optician, who was perplexed at the sudden increase in lens power.

A few months later, I noticed that I had trouble reading. I felt like an older person who can see fine far away but has to ask someone to read the menu options at restaurants. The ophthalmologist prescribed bifocals for me and sent me home.

Contests of who could stare at their nose the longest were popular at the time, and I realized I could not look at my nose with both eyes at the same time. I remember using a red lens I had in my room and placing it over my left eye to see if I could see out of both eyes. I noticed that I saw mostly out of my right eye, and in some parts of my field of vision, I suppressed my left eye's image completely.

I began noticing exotropic strabismic diplopia (double vision from wall-eye) and a wandering outwards of the eyes when observing my eyes at near. The diplopia became more and more frequent, and the two images grew farther and farther apart. Reading was almost impossible. Since I saw two glasses at the same time, I touched the bottle to the glass when pouring liquids to make sure I was pouring inside the glass. (That only took one miss.) Along with double vision, I had no depth perception, and would find myself nearly running into the central metal piece of double doors and streetlights. Sometimes I would try to close my pen and completely miss. When I looked people in the eyes, I saw three eyes (four images, with two superimposed) and two noses.

The ophthalmologist recommended I get strabismus (eye muscle) surgery. Both my parents were shocked at such a drastic option, and my mom reacted by sending me to a series of alternative practitioners. I had several sessions of S.C.E.N.A.R. (Self-Controlled Energo Neuro Adaptive Regulation) in which the doctor would send low levels of electricity to my nerves (specifically my medial and oculomotor nerves) with the hope of stimulating my medial recti (muscles that help my eyes cross) and therefore correcting my exotropia. That treatment just caused a overstimulation of the eye muscles that allow my eyes to turn inwards, in which I would have exotropia in the mornings and evenings, and an esophoria (tendency for the eyes to cross) during the day.

I had my strabismus surgery (bilateral lateral rectus recession) in the beginning of the 8th grade. My eyes then became esotropic, turned inwards ("opposite" eye problem after surgery), and I still had double vision.

Despite this, the surgery was very successful. My exotropic deviation was much less significant. The problems mentioned in the following paragraphs are not complications of the surgery; the strabismus was closely related to other problems that cannot be corrected with strabismus surgery.

For those readers who could spare the technical details, skip this paragraph with the knowledge that my eyes wandered in all directions and were generally confused. I developed a cyclophoria (eyeball "tilt" along the z-axis, which runs through the pupil) and therefore the corresponding torsional diplopia (double vision in which one image appears tilted). Sometimes I had a cramped feeling in my eye muscles, as if my brain could not sort the information correctly, and would tell the wrong muscles (specifically my superior oblique muscles leading to strabismus) to contract when trying to cross my eyes. Other times, I had to juggle three types of double vision (vertical, horizontal, and torsional): when I tried to straighten my eyes in one direction, they would wander in another.

I had convergence insufficiency (my eyes muscles were unable to work together in a way that is required for reading and other close-up work) coupled with accommodation insufficiency (I could not make close objects clear). I had a low AC/A ratio (usually these two functions are proportional; mine was too low). I felt that my school grades would plummet if I did not visit the ophthalmologist soon, so my parents scheduled an appointment with the ophthalmologist.

He prescribed separate distance and reading glasses for me. The lenses were so thick and they made my eyes appear so distorted that people at school used to take them from me and stare at objects an inch away. I remember observing one friend's eyes as she held a dollar bill up to her face, inspecting the smallest details. I would then watch her eyes diverge (wander outwards) as she put on the reading glasses. These glasses were helpful for me; however, they were a crutch to my eyes. I lost the ability to look at objects closer than 20 feet without experiencing double vision and blurriness.

A friend then told me about her brother's eye doctor, Dr. Appelbaum. (Her brother had benefited from vision therapy several years before in the doctor's Bethesda, Maryland, office.) I called him and scheduled an evaluation.

Dr. Appelbaum nailed all the problems at once. He made an immediate connection between the ophthalmologist's various diagnoses. Dr. Appelbaum did not see a pair of eyes entering the exam room; he saw a person entering the room. He recognized that the surgery helped, and my current problems were not complications of the surgery but rather aspects of another problem. He told me that my eye conditions could be helped by changes in diet, posture, office treatment, exercise routines, and attitude. He put what I was experiencing into words, and reassured me that I could learn to better control my vision!

I began my vision therapy treatment in January 2004 and finished in February 2006. I had two to four office sessions per week, took many vacations and several months off from the treatment program, with regular progress evaluations. I worked on being able to accommodate and converge my eyes, being able to converge my eyes with minimal accommodation (increasing my AC/A ratio), as well as training my eyes to track more accurately. My pursuits became smoother over time, my saccades more precise, and my binocularity more and more frequent. I almost never suppressed my left eye's image. While doing my vision therapy exercises, Dr. Appelbaum would answer my questions and provide me with challenges. Now that I no longer go to vision therapy sessions, I no longer have that biweekly stimulation, and I do miss it!

(I admit that I was a patient who actually really looked forward to vision therapy sessions.)

I now have no trouble handling the 11th-grade workload. I can control my eye movements, probably moreso than those who were born with healthy eyes. Other than the very rare exotropic or cyclophoric diplopia, I have achieved stereopsis or depth perception (3-D vision). I can read without having double images or floating words on the page. I can converge my eyes up to about an inch and a half in front of my nose. My eyesight and vision have improved so much that I can read the Snellen Chart all the way down to the last line even without my glasses! I wish I had known about vision therapy sooner. In a perfect world everyone would always be referred for vision therapy whenever the eyes are not straight, experience double vision, attention problems, eyestrain or difficulty reading.

Do You Need Help?

As all of the foregoing chapters have sought to show, doctors specializing in vision therapy are primarily concerned with visual abilities, as well as the impact that good or poor vision has on the whole range of muscular and mental functions. Vision therapy is basically an advanced form of physical training. The visual system is the dominant sensory system, the principal mechanism of control, the one that plays an apparently decisive role in organizing and coordinating all of the various functions of the organism, including the brain.

Dr. A.M. Skeffington, one of the founders of this approach to vision care, once observed that "he who is unstable in his visual world is insecure in his ego." We have shown by reference to selected case histories that this is true, that persons with stressed or seriously deficient visual performance often lack self-confidence and steady nerves, and often manifest undesirable personality traits and patterns of behavior. We have also shown that vision therapy—treating the body/mind system as an essential unit—can produce improvements extending beyond visual scope and acuity to posture, muscular coordination, energy, creative powers, and even to behavior and personality. Effective vision therapy has brought an end not only to blurred vision but also has strengthened intellectual performance and creativity and has changed irritable, complaining personalities with behavior and attention problems into calmer, more achieving, successful, self-confident, men, women and children.

These results are not easily understood or accepted by traditional medicine. And beyond a certain level of generality, they are not easily explainable even by the optometrists who practice vision therapy. No one knows precisely how and why some things happen. There is indeed a certain mystery at the heart of the process. Optometrists are engaged in a fascinating clinical process whose methods and conclusions are being continuously tested and refined by the basic, old-fashioned method of open-minded observation as well as recent double blind, placebo-controlled, multicenter scientific studies. In an age of computers and programmed learning, we all have a tendency to assume that every aspect of life is fully explainable, or should be. We forget that most of today's "hard science" started a number of years ago as someone's clear-eyed observation or intuitive hunch. We fail to remember that every successful creative effort in the history of mankind succeeded because it defied and moved beyond the accepted boundaries of conventional wisdom.

With respect to vision therapy however, there is no need for timidity in the face of conventional doubts. Vision therapy exists and it works. It is apparent that it works because it is soundly grounded in basic truths about the nature of the human organism. We have no doubt at all that a very large number of people in our overstressed society could be relieved of endless headaches, chronic exhaustion, and a whole range of minor ailments and disorders (and even some serious ones) if they were willing and able to undertake a properly defined vision therapy treatment program, resulting in more positive, energetic, and productive lives.

While vision therapy is not yet available widely enough to serve all those who need it, the number of serious and dedicated professional optometrists is steadily growing, and we believe that time and the spreading awareness of its social usefulness will increase public demand and thus lead to its wider availability. It is our earnest hope that this book will play a constructive part in this process.

We close by posing a series of questions, developed in collaboration with several optometrists, that amount to a visual self-evaluation test aimed at helping you determine whether your own (or your child's) visual system is functioning efficiently. If you will consider each question with careful, critical reflection on your own (or your child's) personal situation you should be able to gain a sense of whether you need vision therapy, either to correct a specific visual problem or to alleviate a more general discomforting condition elsewhere in your body that may be related to the way your eyes are functioning.

1. Do you have double vision, see doubled or overlapping words on a page?
2. Do you have headaches while or after doing near vision work?
3. Do words appear to run together when you are reading?

4. Do you fall asleep when reading?
5. Is your seeing and visual work worse at the end of the day?
6. Do you skip or repeat lines when reading?
7. Do you have dizziness or nausea when doing near work?
8. Do you have a head tilt or one eye closed or covered while reading?
9. Do you avoid doing near tasks like reading?
10. Is your reading comprehension low, or does it decline as the day wears on?
11. Do you have trouble keeping your attention centered on reading?
12. Do you not plan or use your time well?
13. Do you often lose your belonging or things?
14. Do you have a hard time driving a car?
15. Does oncoming traffic sometimes appear to be on your side of the road?
16. While driving, do you have a tendency to use the brakes 50 or 60 feet before you come to a stop sign? And do you jam on the brakes at each stop?
17. Do you have any other problems of judging depth when you drive?
18. When you walk, does the horizon appear to move up and down?
19. When you see objects, are they really where they appear to be, or do you often misjudge their true position and sometimes bump into them?
20. Do you avoid sports and games?
21. Do you play tennis, basketball, volleyball, or any other games involving moving balls and players?
22. If you don't, have you ever asked yourself why you don't?
23. Do you have poor, inconsistent performance in sports?
24. If you play games with moving balls, but in a rather clumsy or mediocre way, how do you analyze your shortcomings?
25. In tennis, for example, do you frequently hit the ball on the edge of the racquet or miss it completely?
26. In basketball or baseball, can you pass and catch the ball easily? Can you shoot baskets accurately, or catch a fly ball in center field?
27. How do you rate your eye-brain-hand coordination?
28. Are you disturbed by crowds in theaters, department stores, or shopping centers?
29. Do you avoid frequenting such places?

30. Do you dislike tasks requiring sustained visual concentration?
31. Do you often find yourself distracted, daydreaming, and unusually fatigued after completing a vision task?
32. Do you have tension during close work, and are you a reluctant reader?
33. Are you a slow reader?
34. Can you organize your visual and mental capacities to read and write effectively, or are you disappointed by your performance?
35. Can you accurately reproduce, by drawing or written explanation, what you have just seen?
36. Can you apply these same capacities to solving practical or theoretical problems without the use of pencil and paper? Are you satisfied with your efficiency?
37. If the situation permits or requires, can you read or study for 3 hours or longer without suffering eyestrain and excessive fatigue?
38. Do you experience any lag in seeing clearly when you shift your attention from the television screen across the room, to the book in your hand, or vice versa?
39. Does your stomach bother you after sustained use of your eyes?
40. Are you happy with your overall physical and mental performance? If you are unhappy about this, can you identify the causes, stresses, or blockages that may be responsible for your performing at below your capacity?
41. Do you often forget, or have poor memory?
42. Do you tend to be clumsy, accident prone, or knock things over?
43. Do you have car or motion sickness?

If after pondering these questions, you conclude that vision therapy would help your (or your child's) situation, contact an optometrist who specializes in vision therapy in your neighborhood or town. If you cannot find one with this specialty, show this book to any optometrist, and ask for a referral. If you are not satisfied, contact one of the resources listed in the back of this book for an optometrist specializing in vision therapy. It can improve your (or your child's) vitality, stamina, visual attention, and mental efficiency for a better quality of life.

For more information about vision and vision therapy, contact:

Vision Help Network
www.visionhelp.com
Information on vision therapy and referrals to a doctor specializing in vision therapy.

College of Optometrists in Vision Development (COVD)
www.covd.org
For referrals to a doctor specializing in vision therapy and information on vision therapy.

Optometric Extension Program Foundation
www.oepf.org
Books and materials on vision therapy and referrals to a doctor.

Optometrists Network
www.optometrists.org
Information on vision therapy and referrals to a doctor.

American Optometric Association
www.aoa.org
Information on vision and vision therapy.

Parents Active for Vision Education
www.pavevision.org
Information on vision therapy and referrals to a doctor.

accommodation: The ability of the eye to focus objects at different distances especially at near-point.

acuity: The ability to see clearly and sharply; referred to as eyesight.

ambient visual processing: Guides head, posture, and movement. Helps in perception of depth, motion, brightness, and eye movement control. **Used in peripheral vision.**

amblyopia (lazy eye): A decrease in eyesight of one eye that is not correctable with glasses or contact lenses. It happens when the brain ignores some of the information coming from that eye. Due to a developmental problem, trauma, stress, or a head injury, the lens for the right eye of the glasses **is usually** different than the lens in the left eye of the glasses **in amblyopia.**

anisometropia: When each eye has different refractive powers.

asthenopia: Eyestrain (often with headaches).

astigmatism: A condition **usually** caused by an irregularity in the shape of the cornea (and/or lens) of the eye causing blurred or distorted vision.

bifocal lens: A lens that has two parts, usually the top for distance vision and the bottom for near vision.

binocular vision: The brain's ability to combine images from each eye into one image. When both eyes achieve an identical reinforcing focus on the same object.

cataract: A condition where the lens of the eye begins to become opaque.

ciliary muscle: The muscle attached to the lens **of the eye** that is responsible for the skill of accommodation (focusing).

concave lens: A minus lens whose thinnest portion is in the center; used for nearsightedness or myopia.

cones: The light-sensitive cells in the retina responsible for detail sight and color vision.

conjunctiva: A thin, clear membrane that covers and protects the white portion of the eye (sclera) and the inner portion of the eyelid.

contact lenses: The transparent plastic lenses worn over the corneas of the **eyes instead of glasses** (to correct vision problems.)

convergence: The simultaneous turning **inward** of both eyes that occurs when viewing an approaching object in an effort to maintain binocular vision.

convergence excess: A sensory and neuromuscular anomaly of the binocular visual system characterized by an overconvergence tendency at near.

convergence insufficiency: When the eyes are unable to converge (move toward each other) when looking at a near object. A sensory and neuromuscular anomaly of the binocular vision system, characterized by an inability of the eyes to approach each other, or sustain convergence. **Associated with ADHD.**

convex lens: A plus lens whose thickest portion is in the center; used for farsightedness (hyperopia)

cornea: The transparent, blood-free tissue covering the central front of the eye (over the pupil, iris, and aqueous humor) where initial refraction or bending of light rays occurs as light enters the eye.

cover test: A test of the eyes' alignment in which each eye is covered and then uncovered while their movement is observed.

depth perception: The ability to judge distances by interpreting size, shape, shadows, and overlapping images.

developmental optometry: A branch of optometry that deals with the visual development of children; also referred to as behavioral optometry.

diopter: The unit used to measure the power of a lens.

divergence: The simultaneous turning out of both eyes when viewing an object that is moving away from the eyes.

dominant eye: The eye that a person prefers to use to "sight" objects.

esophoria: The muscle alignment of the two eyes when they have a tendency to turn in toward each other.

esotropia: The inward deviation of the eyes toward each other; known as cross-eyes.

exophoria: The tendency of the eyes to diverge, or turn away from each other.

exotropia: The outward deviation of the eyes from each other.

extraocuclar muscles: The muscles attached to the outside of the eyeball, which control eye movements. Each eye has six muscles.

eyeball: The sense organ of the body that receives light and begins processing it into perceived images.

farsightedness (hyperopia): When light passes through the eye and it focuses behind the retina, resulting in more difficulty with close vision than distance vision.

fixation: The ability of the eyes to attend a stationary target.

fovea: A tiny depression in the center of the retina's macula region where eyesight is best.

fusion: The merging of the images from each eye into a single visual image, which is necessary for appropriate development of binocularity.

glaucoma: An eye disease that occurs when the eye pressure affects the optic nerve; may cause a decrease in visual field.

hypertropia: When one eye is higher than the other.

iris: The colored part of the eye.

lens: The part of the eye responsible for changing its shape so light can focus on the retina.

macula: The **20/20** part of the retina where detailed precise eyesight occurs.

monocular vision: Using only one eye.

nearsightedness (myopia): The inability of the eyes to see objects at a distance.

ophthalmoscope: An instrument used to see the back of the eye.

optic nerve: The bundle of nerve fibers that connect the eye to the brain.

phoropter: An instrument containing many combinations of lenses used to help determine an eyeglass or contact lens prescription.

photophobia: Light sensitivity.

presbyopia: The natural decline of the eye's ability to focus at near distance as a result of normal aging.

prism lens: A lens that bends light in a specific direction; usually used for **eye** muscle problems.

progressive lens: A lens with different prescriptions from the center of the lens to the bottom.

pupil: The black hole in the center of the iris through which light enters the eye.

pursuit eye movements: The ability of the eyes to follow a moving target.

refraction: The determination of lens powers necessary to correct specific amounts of myopia, hyperopia, astigmatism, or presbyopia.

refractive error: Measures the amount of prescription needed so images will appear clearly on the retina.

retina: The light-sensitive tissue in the back of the eye.

retinoscope: An instrument used to measure the bending of light into a person's eye, giving an estimate for prescription glasses.

rods: The light-sensitive cells in the retina that respond to light and dark, movement, and shapes, but not to colors.

saccadic eye movements: The eyes' movement from one target to another.

sclera: The white outer covering of the eye.

sight: The ability of the eyes to discriminate objects; the power of seeing

strabismus: Occurs when one or both eyes turn up, down, inward or outward; when the two eyes do not work together as a team.

20/20 or twenty/twenty: Normal eyesight or visual acuity as measured by the eye doctor's Snellen Eye Chart.

vertical phoria: The tendancy of one eye to look upward rather than to project horizontally in parallel with the other eye.

vertical prism: A lens used to compensate for a vertical imbalance between the eyes.

vertigo: a dizzying sensation of tilting within stable surroundings or of being in tilting or spinning surroundings as a result of a disturbance of some part of the body's balancing mechanism. Caused by medical, inner ear, balance, and vision problems resulting in sensations of motion or spinning that leads to dizziness and discomfort.

vestibular system: A contributor to our balance **system** and our sense of spatial orientation, it is the sensory **system** that provides the dominant input about movement and equilibrioception, and tells us which way is up, which way is down and where an individual is located in space.

vision: The ability to interpret and gain meaning from what is seen utilizing perceptual experiences to form mental images such as a vivid imaginative conception or anticipation.

visual pathway: Nerve impulses take this "road" through the brain from the retina to the optic nerve and beyond to the visual cortex.

yoked prism glasses: are usually prescribed by Behavioral Optometrists skilled in neuro-optometric rehabilitation for patients with visual-spatial midline shift as a result of brain injury, stroke, autism, ADHD, learning difficulties, etc. A wedge of glass or plastic with the thick end called the base and the base ends of the prism positioned in the same direction for each eye used in vision therapy.

Dr. Stan Appelbaum

A graduate of the Illinois College of Optometry, Dr. Stan Appelbaum completed his residency in Optometric Vision Therapy at the State University of New York's College of Optometry in New York City.

He was director of The Vision Therapy Clinic at The Optometric Center of Maryland, Baltimore City Health Department.

Dr. Appelbaum has served as the Maryland State Director of The Optometric Extension Program, an international behavioral vision education and research organization, and he is currently the Maryland State Director/Coordinator and a Fellow of The College of Optometrists in Vision Development, the optometric organization that certifies doctors as specialists in vision therapy.

He has been in private practice with his wife, Barbara Bassin, OTR, BCP for over 20 years in Bethesda and Annapolis, Maryland, combining vision therapy with sensory integration occupational therapy in the same office. He specializes in working with infants, special needs, developmentally delayed, and learning disabled/ADD/ADHD children, adults with visual fatigue/reading difficulties, traumatic brain injury, stroke, and practices functional and developmental concepts in his approach to treating vision problems and enhancing vision skills and abilities. He lectures on topics related to hidden vision problems causing reading problems in bright children, infant vision development, Visual/Vestibular assessment and treatment, visually related learning difficulties, strabismus, amblyopia, the visual demands of computer use, and sports vision.

Southern College of Optometry, in partnership with Dr. Stan Appelbaum, has recently started the first residency program in vision therapy/rehabilitative Optometry in a private practice in Dr. Appelbaum's Bethesda and Annapolis, Maryland offices.

Dr. Appelbaum has served on the Board of Sensory Integration International and the College of Optometrists in Vision Development. He is an Adjunct

Clinical Professor at the Southern College of Optometry and has medical staff privileges at The Shady Grove Adventist Rehabilitation Hospital of Maryland and The National Rehabilitation Hospital in Washington, DC, where he treats patients with visual problems associated with brain injury."

Ann M. Hoopes

Ann M. Hoopes and her husband, Townsend Hoopes, wrote the original *Eye Power* in 1979. The book was immediately published in hard cover by the New York publishing house of Alfred A. Knopf and was widely disseminated and read around the world. For the past 2 decades, it has been in constant demand in soft cover. In more recent years, new information and scientific research results on the positive effects of vision therapy have emerged. Realizing the original book need to be updated, Ann Hoopes joined forces with Dr. Stan Appelbaum to expand *Eye Power* and reintroduce vision therapy to the public.

Born in 1933, Ann Hoopes was raised in Wilmette, Illinois, and Southport, Connecticut, and educated at Wellesley College and the University of Bridgeport. A lifelong advocate of alternative medicine, she founded the first-of-its-kind wellness center, and was an owner of Washington's popular health-food store named, Yes! She still serves on the Board of Dr. James S. Gordon's Center for Mind-Body Medicine.

An accomplished pianist, Ann Hoopes resides in the Washington, DC, area, where she has served on the National Symphony Board and for decades produced musicals for a local amateur group, appropriately named "The Hoopes Troops." An active member of both The Chevy Chase Club (in Maryland) and The Country Club of Fairfield (in Connecticut), she is recognized as an outstanding athlete even at her advancing age. A widow with five children and nine grandchildren, she maintains offshore properties on the island of Barbuda in the British West Indies and at Vilcabamba, Ecuador.

accommodation (focusing), 137, 149

Adderal and ADHD, 15

ADHD or vision problems, 1, 2, 3, 8, 10, 13, 14, 15-26

ADHD and Convergence Insufficiency (CI), 4, 14, 19, 20, 31-32

amblyopia (lazy eye), 7, 25, 32, 33, 42, 44, 52, 58, 80, 98, 149, 155

anisometropia, 111, 149

Appelbaum, Dr. Bryce, 89, 90, 126,

artistic skill and visual defects, 13

astigmatism, 53, 56, 64, 111, 138

Autism, 8, 39-50, 94

recovering from, 63, 127

Autism Speaks, 49

autism and vision problems, 1, 2, 3, 8, 10, 13, 14, 16, 17, 18, 22, 27, 28, 29, 30, 35, 39, 40, 42, 44, 45, 46, 49, 53, 63, 69, 71, 72, 73, 74, 75, 77

baiance problems, 8, 74, 78, 81

balance rail activity, 121

Barry, Dr. Sue, 52

Bassin, OTR, Barbara, 4, 48, 49, 155

Bates, Dr William, 52, 132

Baxstrom, Dr. Curtis, 28

behavioral optometry, 150

behavior problems and vision, 42, 134

bifocals, 21, 25, 37, 116, 139,

bilateral motor equivalents activity, 105, 120, 122

Birnbaum, Dr. Marty, 54

Binocular Fusion Flexibility, 19

Binocular Stamina, 19

body awareness procedures, 60, 98, 99, 100, 103, 104, 105, 106, 120, 121

Brinkley, Douglas, v

Burns, Dr. Carole, 94, 96

calisthenics in vision therapy, 54

car sickness and vision therapy, 102

Chiropractic manipulation, 69

Cohen, MD, Philip J, vii

Checklist of Vision Problems, 144-146

College of Optometrists in Vision Development (COVD), xi

compensatory adaptation of body/ mind system, 10

computer processes and eye-brain functions, 145

see also cybernetics

clumsiness, 46, 49, 112

Concerta and ADHD, 15

Convergence Insufficiency (CI), and ADHD, 4, 14, 19, 20, 31-32

concentration problems and vision, xii

corneal refractive therapy, 95-96

creativity and vision, 70, 143

cross-eyed, see strabismus

Defeat Autism Now (DAN), 49

depth perception, 7–8, 18–19, 21, 42, 43, 46–47, 52, 58, 61, 66, 79, 93–96, 127–128, 139, 142, 150 developmental optometry, 3, 10, 12, 24, 30–31, 39, 44–45, 47, 59, 111, 117, 135, 150

depression and vision problems, 66, 73, 103, 106

detail, perception of, 24, 71, 79, 82, 98, 107, 108, 128, 149

Dexedrine and ADHD, 15

diagnosis of visual problems, 8, 9, 10, 13, 22, 30, 31, 33, 40, 44, 52, 71, 74, 78, 84, 99, 105, 135, 137, 156

distance vision, cultural influences on, 55, 62, 64, 86, 100, 101, 113, 114, 149, 151

dizziness and vision problems, 8, 21, 62, 71, 74, 76, 78, 81, 102, 145, 154

double vision, 8, 12, 19, 21–22, 31–32, 34, 46, 57–58, 64, 71–72, 74, 76–78, 81, 83–84, 87, 137, 139, 140–142, 144

Draisin, Dr. Neil, 53,

dry eye, 86

Dyslexia and Vision Problems, 27

dyslexia symptoms and eye coordination, 3, 27, 30, 33, 36

esophoria, 46, 64, 140, 151

esotropia, 151

Etting, Dr. Gary, 31, 91
   to increase visual space intake, 100, 107
   for size constancy perception, 98, 107

walking, 3, 6, 21, 39, 42, 46, 47, 54, 55, 66, 76, 79, 80, 81, 121, 122

eye aerobics, 33, 131, 132

eye muscles, test of, 1, 10, 57, 84, 119, 126, 131, 132, 140,

eye-brain connection, 145

eye control, 19

eye drops, 44,

eye movement disorders, 11, 12, 34, 43, 66, 149

eye tracking disorders, 93

eye patches, 6

eyesight and vision, 1, 142

eye tests, 40

farsightedness, *see* hyperopia

fatigue, chronic, and vision problems, 8, 18, 19, 30, 34, 43, 58, 59, 62, 64, 65, 79, 132, 146, 155

feedback process in vision, 72

fidgeting, 1, 3,

field of vision, enlargement of, 10, 85, 86, 106, 107, 108, 109, 110, 113, 117, 122, 123, 124, 125, 127, 129, 139

Fitzgerald, Larry, 91
   accommodation, 137
   binocular, problems with, 12

Focus Stamina, 19

Fortenbacher, Dr. Dan, vii, 33

Friedman, Dr. Henry M., 99

Getman, Dr. G. N., 54

Gesell, Dr. Arnold, 27

Gianutsos, Dr. Rosalind, 79

glare, effects of, 95,

glasses, 7, 18, 21, 24, 32, 35, 36, 43, 44, 45, 52, 53, 54, 55, 56, 57, 61, 62, 64, 69, 76, 82, 83, 84, 85, 86, 87, 96, 100, 101, 110, 114, 116, 117, 135, 137, 138, 139, 141, 142, 149, 150, 153, 154

goal-oriented vision therapy, 99

Gordon, MD, James, v

hand-eye coordination, 37, 127

Handwriting Without Tears, 123

Harmon, Dr. Darrell Boyd, 114, 68

headaches and visual problems, 1, 4, 8, 9, 12, 18, 21, 22, 31, 57, 58, 61, 62, 64, 65, 68, 78, 79, 81, 83, 116, 117, 132, 144, 149

Hemianopsia, 85

Hilgartner, Dr. Pete, 63

Hillier, Dr. Carl, 51, 52, 57, 92

Hong, Dr. Carole, 9

hyperactivity, 1, 15, 18, 63, 94, 115, 124

hyperopia, 111, 137, 138, 150, 151, 153

hypertropia, 115, 116, 152

Infinity Walk Procedure, 134–135

jogging in a vision therapy program, 54

Johnson, Lucy Nugent, 7

Kaplan, Dr. Mel, 39

Kawar, OTR Mary, 47, 51, 132, 133

Lazy eye, (amblyopia), xii, 7, 19, 25, 32, 33, 44, 52, 58, 80, 98, 149

Learning process, 105

Learning Disabilities and Vision Problems, 27

    space/time relationships in, 10, 127, 128,

Lemer, Patricia, 9, 48

lenses, xii, 1, 4–5, 7, 9–11, 13–14, 21, 24–25, 32, 34–36, 40, 43–45, 52, 56–57, 62, 67–71, 74, 79, 81, 82–86, 92–93, 95–96, 98, 101–102, 106, 109–112, 114–117, 119, 135, 138, 141, 149, 150, 152

    bifocal, 21, 25, 36, 37, 100, 116, 139, 149

    compensatory, 82, 109, 111, 116

    corrective, 1, 13, 14, 70, 104, 109, 112, 138

    contact, see contact lenses

    developmental, x, 3, 5, 7–8, 10, 11–13, 24, 30–31, 35, 39–40, 42, 43–45, 47–48, 59, 76, 109, 111–112, 117, 135, 149–150, 155,

    minus, 109, 110, 150

    for myopia, 7, 60, 107, 110, 111, 112, 113, 114, 150, 152, 153

    low plus, 100, 106, 114, 115

    polaroid, 116

    preventive, 99, 112

prisms, xii, 6, 7, 45, 71, 72, 74, 79, 81, 82, 83, 84, 85, 86, 87, 98
rehabilitative, 8, 79, 83, 86, 155
stress-reducing, 11, 34, 36, 43, 93, 106
therapeutic, 5, 9, 24, 48, 68, 79, 81, 82, 84, 102, 106, 109, 111, 112, 115, 116–117
Lenses, Stress-Reducing, 1, 34, 36, 43, 93, 106
Low Vision, 14, 83, 86
Lowe, Dr. Sue, 90, 101

McDonald, Dr. Larry, 133
Marsden Ball Technique, 130
Mazer, Dr. Harvey, 35
minus lenses, 109, 110
motion sickness and vision therapy, 102, 146
Multiple Sclerosis, 77
myopia, 7, 60, 107, 110, 111, 112, 113, 114, 150, 152, 153, 158
cultural influences on, lenses for, 34, 43, 56, 69, 86, 106, 110, 111, 114, and near-point visual stress, 66
lens therapy, 35, 109,

near-point visual stress, 66,
nearsightedness, *see* myopia, 7, 42, 69, 95, 107, 111, 112, 113, 116, 138, 150, 152

neck pain and visual problems, 8, 9, 10, 13, 22, 30, 31, 33, 40, 44, 52, 71, 74, 78, 84, 99, 103, 135, 137, 156,
nervous system, "lead system" of, 9, 40, 45, 72, 77, 99, 106, 111, 132
Neuro-Optometric Rehabilitation, 83
Neurological Vision Problems, 83
nutrition, 6, 8, 49, 68, 69, 89

objects
perception of, 24, 71, 79, 82, 98, 107, 108, 128, 149
Oculomotor skills, 35, 78, 96, 139
eye movement control, 34, 43, 66, 149
Occupational Therapy, 33, 41, 46, 47, 48, 82, 83, 116, 123, 135, 155
combined with vision therapy, 48, 49
Optometric Extension Program Foundation, 147
Optometrist, role of in vision therapy, vi, ix, xi, xii, 3, 5, 8, 9, 10, 12, 13, 14, 23, 24, 30, 31, 39, 44, 45, 49, 52, 54, 59, 62, 69, 70, 71, 74, 75, 78, 81, 91, 92, 93, 94, 97, 98, 99, 100, 103, 107, 109, 110, 111, 112, 115, 117, 119, 121, 125, 128, 137, 143, 144, 146, 147, 154, 155
Orthokeratology, 95-96
Osteopathic Physicians, 106
Osteopathic treatment, 69

Padula, Dr. Bill, 78, 79
patching, 32, 71
Parents Active in Vision Education
(PAVE) xi, 66
pencil and straw exercise, 107, 123,
128
perception, 1, 3, 7, 8, 18, 19, 20, 21,
24, 42, 43, 46, 47, 52, 58, 59, 61,
66, 71, 72, 73, 79, 82, 93, 94, 95,
96, 98, 103, 107, 108, 110, 121,
127, 128, 139, 142, 149, 150
constriction of, as reaction to
stress, 114
peripheral vision, 19
peripheral vision expansion, 133
peripheral vision problems, 19, 43,
47, 54, 93, 107, 108, 109, 114,
124, 125, 133, 134, 149
and myopia, 7, 60, 107, 110,
111, 112, 113, 114, 150, 152,
153, 158
personality development and vision,
97
Pervasive Developmental Disorders
(PDD), 40
physical therapy, 8, 9, 76, 80, 83, 97
plus lenses, 106, 110, 114, 115
polaroid lenses, 116
Politzer, Dr. Thomas, 72
posture, 6, 8, 10, 32, 34, 42, 45, 46,
51, 54, 55, 60, 67, 68, 69, 70, 76,
79, 80, 82, 83, 100, 105, 106, 107,
111, 120, 121, 124, 129, 131, 138,
141, 143, 149
Post Trauma Vision Syndrome

(PTVS), 78, 79, 80
Press, Dr. Leonard vi, xiii, 98
preventive lenses, see lenses,
developmental
prisms, use of, in vision therapy, xii,
6, 7, 45, 71, 72, 74, 79, 81, 82, 83,
84, 85, 86, 87, 98
problem solving and vision, 114
psychological effects of visual
deficiencies, see personality
development and vision
reading difficulties, 81, 155
field of vision, 10, 84, 85, 86,
106, 107, 108, 109, 110, 113,
117, 122, 123, 124, 125, 127,
129, 139
vision problems, 1, 2, 3, 8, 10,
13, 14, 16, 17, 18, 22, 27, 28,
29, 30, 35, 39, 40, 42, 44, 45,
46, 49, 53, 63, 69, 71, 72, 73,
74, 75, 77, 90, 101, 102, 109,
150, 154, 155
PTA, National Parents and Teachers
Association Resolution on
Learning-Related Vision Problems,
30

Renshaw, Dr. Samual, 5
retinoscope, use of, 60, 153
Reversals and Vision Problems, 30
Ritalin aand ADHD, 15

Saccadic eye movements, 153
Sanet, Dr. Robert, 8
Scheiman, Dr. Mitchell, 4

Sensory Integration Therapy, combined with Vision Therapy, 47, 48. 49
side vision, test of, 109, 133
See also peripheral vision Problems
Schulman, Dr. Randy, 44
Size constancy perception, 98, 107, 108, 128, 129
Skeffington, Dr. A. M., 51, 121, 143
Snellen eye test, 13, 29, 138, 142, 153
Space, visual intake of, 100
space/time relationships in vision, 10
sports and vision therapy, 89
sports visual skills, 92-93
standing awareness procedure,105–106, 121
stereopsis, *see* depth perception
strabismus, v, 4, 7, 20, 33, 36, 42, 44, 52, 58, 78, 80, 111–112, 115, 139–140, 153, 155
developmental lenses for, 112
esotropia, 151
exotropia, 139–140, 151
surgery vs. vision therapy, 33, 93, 95
Strattera and ADHD, 15
Stress and Vision Problems, 59-60
stress-reducing lenses, 114
String Procedure (Brock String), 108, 128, 129
Stroke, 71-86

structural approach to visual defects, 13
Suchoff, Dr. Irwin, 75
Sunbeck, Dr. Deborah, 133
Sunglasses, use of, 59
Swimming in vision therapy programs, 54
Symbolizing nature of vision, 113

tactile defensiveness, 47, 48
taking in more visual space, 82, 126, 133
Tannen, Dr. Barry, viii, 30
Thumb Pursuits exercise, 107, 123, 127, 130
toe walking, 43
Torgerson, Dr. Nancy, vii, 6, 29, 36
training lenses, use of, 101
transitions in vision therapy, 55
Traumatic Brain Injury (TBI), 71-86
visual symptoms of TBI, 78, 81
tunnel vision, 60
See also peripheral vision
Two Sticks activity, 107, 123, 127, 128
vertical phoria, 100, 101, 153
vertigo and vision problems, 8, 62, 78, 81, 102, 154
vestibular problems and visual processing, 10, 35, 52, 71, 79, 83, 90, 114
Vicci, Dr. Vincent, 74

vision as body/mind "lead system,", 10, 13, 99, 103, 105, 108, 112, 121, 123, 143,

2009 Super Bowl, 91

classroom, 2, 28, 30,34, 35, 46, 91, 123, 135, 155

Checklist of Vision Problems, 144-146

combined with Occupational Therapy, 13, 41, 46, 47, 48, 82, 83, 116

home procedures in, 32, 44, 82, 97–98, 123, 130

physical conditioning exercises in, 54, 55, 103

transitions, *see* transitions in vision therapy

Visual Field Loss, 84, 85

vision therapy, definition, 4

visual hygiene, 35, 66, 68

Visual Midline Shift Syndrome (VMSS), 78, 79, 80,

visual perception, 1, 3, 20, 58, 59, 73, 79, 103, 121

Visual Information Processing, 20

visual processing, 10, 35, 52, 71, 79, 83, 90, 114, 149

Visual Tracking, 19

visualization, 20, 59, 93, 94

Visual-Vestibular connection, 10, 35, 52, 71, 79, 83, 90, 114

carsickness, motion sickness, and vision problems, 32, 62 , 71, 102,

walking, role in vision therapy, 3, 6, 21, 39, 42, 46, 47, 54, 55, 66, 76, 79, 80, 81, 121, 122
techniques for,

Wisneski MD, Leonard, vi

Wolff Wand activity, 107, 123, 125, 127, 130

Wright, Dr. Mark, 22

Yoked prisms (ambient lenses), 45, 81, 82, 83, 85

7812917R0

Made in the USA
Charleston, SC
11 April 2011